User Experience Research and Usability of Health Information Technology

Health information technology (HIT) is a critical component of the modern healthcare system. Yet to be effective and safely implemented in healthcare organizations and physicians and patients' lives, it must be usable and useful. User Experience (UX) research is required throughout the full system design lifecycle of HIT products, which involve a user-centered and human-centered approach. This book discusses UX research frameworks, study designs, methods, data-analysis techniques, and a variety of data collection instruments and tools that can be used to conduct UX research in the healthcare space, all of which involve HIT and digital health. This book is for academics and scholars to be used to design studies for graduate dissertation work, in independent research, or as a textbook for UX/usability courses in health informatics or related health information and communication courses. This book is also useful for UX practitioners because it provides guidance on how to design a user research or usability study and focuses on leveraging a mixed-methods approach, including step-by-step by instructions and best practices for conducting:

- Field studies
- Interviews
- Focus groups
- Diary studies
- Surveys
- Heuristic evaluations
- Cognitive walkthroughs
- Thinking aloud

A plethora of standardized surveys and retrospective questionnaires (SUS, Post-study System Usability Questionnaire (PSSUQ)) are also included. UX researchers and healthcare professionals will gain an understanding of how to design a rigorous, yet feasible study that generates useful insights to inform the design of usable HIT. Everything from consent forms to how many participants to include in a usability study has been covered in this book. The author encourages user-centered design (UCD), mixed-methods, and collaboration among interdisciplinary teams. Knowledge from many interrelated disciplines, such as psychology, technical communication (TC), and human–computer interaction (HCI), together with experiential knowledge from experts is offered throughout the text.

Jessica Lynn Campbell has a PhD in Philosophy, and a master's degree in English—Technical Communication, both of which she earned from the University of Central Florida (UCF). She is an experienced, expert UX researcher and designer, and technical communication practitioner, having held various roles in the healthcare and health informatics space creating content, engaging in digital marketing, and performing UX research for product and service development. Simultaneously with her industry career, Jessica holds an educator role. As a professor of English, she teaches several technical communication and UX courses. Her expertise and research interests intersect the technical communication, HCI, and UX disciplines where she focuses on the usability of health information technology (HIT) and leveraging user-centered design (UCD) and equity design to research and design HIT for various audiences. She has experience conducting mixed-method studies, including both quantitative and qualitative methods in investigations of the usability of telemedicine and similar digital health interventions. In addition to her research interest in the healthcare space, Jessica's scholarly and academic interests include a broad scope of technical and professional communication (TPC) pedagogy, particularly exploring the engagement of students in social justice work, solving wicked problems, and improving digital literacy. She is curious, eager to collaborate, and contributes to the TPC community to continue to expand the TPC discipline.

User Experience Research and Usability of Health Information Technology

Jessica Lynn Campbell, PhD

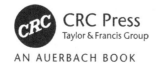

CRC Press
Taylor & Francis Group

AN AUERBACH BOOK

First edition published 2024
2385 NW Executive Center Drive, Suite 320, Boca Raton FL 33431

and by CRC Press
4 Park Square, Milton Park, Abingdon, Oxon, OX14 4RN

CRC Press is an imprint of Taylor & Francis Group, LLC

© 2024 Taylor & Francis Group, LLC

ISBN: 9781032608785 (hbk)
ISBN: 9781032162768 (pbk)
ISBN: 9781003460886 (ebk)

DOI: 10.1201/9781003460886

Typeset in Garamond
by Newgen Publishing UK

Contents

Illustrations

FIGURES

TABLES

Abbreviations

ADR	adverse drug reaction
AHLTA	Armed forces Health Longitudinal Technology Application
AOI	area of interest
ARRA	American Recovery and Reinvestment Act
ASQ	After-Scenario Questionnaire
ATT	attractiveness
CCDSS	Consumer-oriented Clinical Decision Support System
CDS	clinical decision support
CDSS	clinical decision support system
CHIS	clinical/consumer health information system
CPOE	computerized physician order entry [system]
CSQ	Client Satisfaction Questionnaire
CSUQ	Computer Usability Satisfaction Survey
CT	Computer Tomography
CUSI	Computer User Satisfaction Inventory
DSS	decision support system
DTC	direct-to-consumer
ED	emergency department
EF	effectiveness
eHEALS	eHealth Literacy Scale
EHR	electronic health record
ER	Expectation Ratings
EUCS	End-User Computer Satisfaction
GOMS	goals, operators, methods, and selection rules
GP	general practitioner
HCD	human-centered design
HCI	human–computer interaction
Health-ITUES	Health Information Technology Usability Evaluation Scale
HINTS	Health Information National Trends Survey
HIS	health information system
HIT	health information technology

HITECH	Health Information Technology for Economic and Clinical Health Act of 2009
HQ-I	hedonic quality: identity
HQ-S	hedonic quality: simulation
IAA	interannotator agreement
ICU	intensive care unit
ID	Identification Information
ISO	International Organization of Standardization
KLM	keystroke-level modeling (KLM)
meCUE	Modular Evaluation of Components of User Experience
mHealth	mobile health
MWL	mental workload
NASA-TLX	NASA-Task Load Index
NIH	National Institutes of Health
NIHR	National Institute for Health Research
NIST	National Institute of Standards and Technology
NPS	Net Promotor Score
ONC	Office of the National Coordinator for Health Information Technology
PACT	Patient Assessment of Communication During Telemedicine
PHI	personal health information
PHR	personal health records
PIMS	Personal Innovativeness Toward Mobile Services
POR	point of regard
PQ	pragmatic quality
PSSUQ	Post-Study System Usability Questionnaire
PTIDB	Perceived Telemedicine Importance, Disadvantages, and Barriers
PUTQ	Purdue Usability Questionnaire
QDAS	qualitative data analysis software
QUIS	Questionnaire for User Interface Satisfaction
ROI	return on investment
SCS	System Causability Scale
SEQ	Single Ease Question
SIS	Surgical Information Systems
SME	subject matter expert
SMEQ	Subject Mental Effort Question

SUMI	Software Usability Measurement Inventory
SUS	System Usability Scale
SUTAQ	Service User Technology Acceptability Questionnaire
T2D	type 2 diabetes
TAM	technology acceptance model
TC	technical communication
TIUQ	Telemedicine Interface Usability Questionnaire
TMPQ	Telemedicine Perception Questionnaire
TSQ	Telemedicine Satisfaction Questionnaire
TSUQ	Telemedicine Satisfaction and Usefulness Questionnaire
TUQ	Telehealth Usability Questionnaire
U&G	uses and gratifications [framework]
UCD	user-centered design
UE	usability engineering
UEQ	User Experience Questionnaire
UI	user interface
UIM	Usability Inspection Methods (UIMs)
UME	Usability Magnitude Estimation
UMUX	Usability Metric for User Experience
USE	Usefulness, Satisfaction, and Ease of Use
UX	user experience
WD	withdrawal
WIMT	wireless internet services via mobile technology

Acknowledgments

This book was conceived partially from my graduate student experience designing my dissertation study and conducting a lengthy, comprehensive literature review to prepare for it, but also through the many conversations I had with colleagues at conferences and during our Building Digital Literacy (BDL) collaborative meetings, set-up by Dr. Ann Hill Duin and Dr. Isabel Pedersen. The BDL collaborators include Dr. Jason Tham, Dr. Daniel Hocutt, Dr. Mollie Stambler, and many other important scholars in Technical and Professional Communication (TPC) and related disciplines. Our BDL meetings and thoughtful conversations all shed light on the content and framework for this text. To all those in the BDL collaborative and those I have engaged with academically through mutual scholarship, I thank you. I also want to thank Dr. David Katan, who I met and partnered with through the Trans-Atlantic and Pacific Project (TAPP). Our many conversations regarding translation considerations, user-centered design, and the real-world translation projects we implemented in our courses has inspired and illuminated the numerous problems in, and solutions regarding, the user-centered design of information for an international audience.

I want to thank the reviewers of my manuscript for the time and expertise they leveraged to critically review my proposal and provide valuable feedback that guided the scope of the book and informed my thinking of the theoretical and practical information I included. Dr. Kirk St. Amant and Dr. Janice (Ginny) Redish offered insight from their technical communication scholarship, particularly regarding intercultural communication and industry practices. I thank Dr. Andre W. Kushniruk and Dr. Elizabeth M. Borycki, whose continuous human factors research of health information technology (HIT) has contributed greatly to my knowledge and expertise and whose many studies are cited in this book.

I want to extend my huge thanks and gratitude to Dr. Jeff Sauro and Dr. James (Jim) R. Lewis. Not only have their numerous studies been used as evidence to support research design considerations in this text and in my past academic and industry scholarship, but their ongoing personal communication with me contributed greatly to this book. In particular, when trying to synthesize the scientific literature on quantitative methods and sample population size, Jeff was extremely helpful and responsive to my many questions by providing details and resources to support the recommendations provided in this book. I am so grateful for Jeff and Jim's research, the ongoing support and communication they offered to me as a scholar and professional UX researcher, and their MeasuringU website and usability information and the tools they provided.

This book was also heavily influenced by my industry experience in marketing, content management, technical communication, and user experience (UX) research and design. Observing the gaps in knowledge between rigorous, scholarly UX research and the studies executed in everyday practice in the field boosted my aspiration to write this book and heavily influenced its content. Lori Hawkins, who I have had the honor of being led by, the privilege of being taught by, and the pleasure of collaborating with, has delightfully offered her wisdom and guidance. Lori created a comfortable space and steadfast team that has allowed creativity to flourish. She has certainly influenced my career and the accomplishments I have been able to achieve, one being writing this book. Other influential figures inspired me and afforded me the ability to both practice in my discipline and learn new skills. Both Richard Milan and Bethany Schenk are leaders who are emersed in their business and hold a great deal of knowledge of business, sales, marketing, technology, productivity, resourcefulness, utility, and interpersonal communication and collaboration. I learned so much from working in environments guided by great leaders like Richard and Bethany. Thank you!

Lastly, I always want to acknowledge and thank my family whose support, encouragement, and love are consistent, continuous, and unconditional. I am privileged to have parents who allowed me to be creative, to get dirty (figuratively and literally), explore opportunities, fail and succeed, and provide gentle guidance and support along the way. I would not be where I am today without my family. I love you with all of my heart.

1

Introduction

This chapter provides an overview of the modern-day healthcare landscape to provide context for how health information technology (HIT) is deployed, used, and relied upon for the dissemination of health information, delivery of healthcare, and production of specific health outcomes, among other implications. The significance of usability studies of HIT is increasingly being recognized and advocated for by academics, health professionals, and even federal bodies, such as the U.S. National Institute of Standards and Technology (NIST) (Schumacher & Lowry, 2010; ONC, 2012). The chapter ends with a brief discussion of how the book is organized and a description of each chapter.

THE IMPORTANCE OF HEALTH INFORMATION TECHNOLOGY

Information technology is increasingly being used in the healthcare sector. HIT can also be referred to using the broad term "eHealth," which encompasses a wide variety of technologies that facilitate healthcare, health information exchange, and electronic communication among health providers, patients, and other stakeholders (Sousa & Lopez, 2017). As such, HIT is a primary subject of scholarly, practitioner, and healthcare professional interest. HIT is used to facilitate healthcare delivery, such as telemedicine (Bashshur, 1995; de Souza et al., 2017). Mobile health applications (mHealth) are used to support patients' disease management (Sarkar et al., 2016) and/or to promote personal health tracking or behavior modifications to improve health (Islam et al., 2020). Electronic health records (EHRs) or personal health records (PHRs) summarize patient health statuses and support cross-organizational collaboration between physicians and communication between physicians and patients (Horsky &

DOI: 10.1201/9781003460886-1

Ramelson, 2016; Kaipio et al., 2017; Monkman & Kushniruk, 2013b; Sandefer et al., 2015). Clinical/consumer health information systems (CHIS), decision support systems (DSS), and other Computerized Physician Order Entry systems (CPOEs) are other forms of HIT that support physicians in making diagnoses, offering treatment options, and dispensing pharmaceuticals (Kushniruk, 2001; Main et al., 2010; Press et al., 2015). Telemedicine is an alternative medical care option, whereby medical consultation, diagnosis, and treatment are delivered via telecommunication technologies (Bashshur, 1995). Direct-to-consumer (DTC) telemedicine is available to the public as a healthcare delivery option for patients to gain access to healthcare remotely or virtually (Uscher-Pines et al., 2015). Likewise, numerous health providers provision health information and messages and market their services to the public through digital communication methods, such as online portals, health information websites, and other consumer-facing platforms. A large, multifaceted, multilingual diversity of users access eHealth to learn about specific health conditions and healthcare options, manage their health, be able to perform behaviors that lead to improved health, and make health-related decisions (Bodie & Dutta, 2008; Maramba, et al., 2019).

The U.S. National Institute for Health Research (NIHR) defines health technologies or health IT as "all interventions used to promote health, prevent and treat disease, and improve rehabilitation and long-term care" (Hung et al, 2013; Main et al., 2010, p. G). Similarly, Alotaibi and Federico (2017) refer to HIT as the application of information processing hardware and software to store, retrieve, share, and use healthcare information, data, and knowledge for communication and decision-making. Likewise, this book adheres to the broadest definition of HIT, casting a wide net to include the many applications of technology in the healthcare sector and to be able to provide many examples of different ways of evaluating and understanding the usability of HIT.

HIT Usability Requirement

The impetus for HIT to be usable is imperative and essential for the safe use and utilization of HIT, as well as to increase the acceptance and adoption of HIT. Therefore, usability studies of HIT are critical during the beginning, middle, and late stages of the design of HIT, as well as subsequent to its implementation or final product release. In addition, the continuous evaluation of HIT usability is needed as health and healthcare delivery is dynamic and context-dependent; it therefore requires continuous investigation to ensure it is being used by the individuals it is designed for in safe, effective, and meaningful ways. U.S. federal legislation even requires HIT, like EHR, to be developed for usability and implemented to achieve meaningful use by the intended users (HITECH, 2009; ONC, 2012).

PURPOSE OF THIS BOOK

The purpose of this book is to provide researchers, technical communicators, health information designers and developers, practitioners, and clinicians with a guide to designing and conducting usability studies of HIT that will provide valuable insight and useful findings to allow for improvements to be made in the usability of the HIT under investigation. This book encourages iterative design practices and user-centered design (UCD) that calls for all stakeholders to be involved in the full system design lifecycle—from understanding the target users and technology specifications, to conducting usability testing, to making design modifications, to full implementation of the final product or system, and finally conducting validation testing to ensure the product is usable and useful (Høstgaard et al., 2011; Kushniruk & Patel, 2004; Lyles et al., 2014).

Designing and delivering usable digital texts and applications is a central aim in the digital world. Good usability has the power to change human behavior, promote the acceptance of products and services (Davis, 1989; Hibbard & Peters, 2003; Kushniruk, 2001; Sandefer et al., 2015), and shape the user experience (Norman, 1988). The healthcare domain is no exception to the usability rule. Designing usable HIT is a key initiative in the healthcare industry because it is integral to modern healthcare systems and aligns with the patient-centered healthcare paradigm (Eysenbach, 2000; Tuckson & Hodgkins, 2017). Health information technology (HIT) promises to improve the delivery, quality, access, and experience of healthcare, and ultimately improve worldwide health; however, despite the affordances offered by HIT, poor usability has been a major barrier to its widespread acceptance and adoption (Kushniruk & Patel, 2004; Kushniruk et al., 2008; Sousa & Lopez, 2017). UCD and usability testing of HIT during the iterative design process is an effective method of designing and delivering usable HIT (Kinzie et al., 2002; Peute & Jaspers, 2007; Peute et al., 2015b). The aim of this book is to drive the momentum and motivation to perform mixed-methods usability studies of HIT.

Who Is This Book For?

This book has a very wide intended audience. First, it is for health information UX researchers, designers, and providers; healthcare professionals; and technical communicators who work in the healthcare field, for whom it can act as a field guide to design and conduct usability studies using a mixture of and multiple methods. These stakeholders hold the power to design and deliver usable HIT that ultimately improve healthcare delivery and health outcomes. Mixed-methods is the leverage of more than one method of evaluating usability, and can be considered a pluralistic framework for conducting usability investigations. Researchers are encouraged to select the best method that allows them to answer their research question or obtain the insight they desire in order to design and deliver usable health technology products. Using mixed-methods affords a large, rich data corpus (because you are using many methods to obtain different sets of data) and enables data triangulation (comparing two data sets to corroborate or contradict findings) to be performed. Mixed-methods offers a more comprehensive understanding of usability, and the limitations of any one method may be offset by the affordances of another method.

This book is also written for scholars, academics, instructors, and graduate students to use as a reference manual, course textbook, or research tool, as it is filled with practical and tactic knowledge regarding usability engineering and UCD applied in the healthcare sector. Several universities offer health communication, medical writing, and health informatics courses that involve various aspects of human–computer interaction (HCI). Thus, this book serves as a textbook to educate on the human factors involved in the usability of HIT, and it can be used by graduate students whose research interests intersect health informatics, HCI, and technical communication to help in the design and completion of a dissertation research study.

ORGANIZATION OF THE BOOK

This book is divided into several parts that follow the UCD stages and discuss the types of formative and summative usability testing that are conducted in each stage of the UCD process. In this fashion, readers are able to follow the book as a guide while performing UCD and learn about the types of methods that are most appropriately applied during the stages of UCD, as well as which methods afford the discovery of valuable insight that can be used to improve the usability of HIT.

- *Chapter 1: Introduction.* This introductory chapter broadly defines HIT and the impetus for performing mixed-methods usability studies of HIT. It also provides an overview of what information will be presented in the book and how the book is organized. This introductory chapter provides evidence for the exigency of usable HIT in today's modern, digitalized society.
- *Chapter 2: Definitions: Usability, UX, and UCD.* This chapter offers many definitions of usability that have been developed and used in the fields of technical communication, HCI, and UX. Usefulness is discussed is an independent variable, but is required for HIT adoption by users. The implications of usability on the user experience are also discussed. Lastly, the user-centered design (UCD) process is described as an iterative design lifecycle that includes all stakeholders (clinicians, patients, researchers, etc.). This chapter also touches upon the next chapters on individual and contextual determinants of usability and the various usability testing methods that are used in the formative and summative stages of UCD/ full-system design lifecycle.
- *Chapter 3: Audience Analysis: Individual and Contextual Usability Determinants.* This chapter discusses the multidimensional factors that affect usability by distinguishing individual/subjective and contextual/ external factors: knowledge of cognitive, social, physical, environmental, etc. This chapter explains formative and summative usability testing and what methods are used for each type, as well as the stage of the UCD process in which each testing method occurs.
- *Chapter 4: Quantitative and Qualitative Methods.* This chapter defines and explains quantitative and qualitative methods, what type of data is obtained from using each method, how it is analyzed, and what can be concluded or inferred from each method.
- *Chapter 5: Mixed-methods Study Design and Rigor.* This chapter asserts mixed-methods to be a beneficial approach to conducting comprehensive and valuable usability studies of health information technology. It informs researchers how to approach designing a mixed-methods study by first identifying their object of inquiry (what technology are they studying) and what they want to discover about usability (develop their research questions). They can then select the best methods, as explained in the subsequent chapters. The chapter discusses the affordances (rich data corpus,

greater interaction with data, more usability metrics able to be measured) and limitations (resource-intensive, costly, timely) of employing mixed-methods. Lastly, the chapter discusses how scientific studies are considered rigorous and how the quality of one's study is evaluated differently depending on whether the study is quantitative or qualitative. The criteria for evaluating the rigor of one's study will be defined including general-izability, validity, and fidelity. An explanation of data triangulation and feasibility is also included in this chapter.

- *Chapter 6: Content Analysis.* This describes the content analysis research methodology, and offers various coding techniques and ways to approach making sense of a wide variety of qualitative data, including using a frame-work approach, inductive coding, or an a priori coding scheme. Content analysis is a method used to discover what type of health communications exist, which helps to explicate the problem with existing technology, lack of usable technology, or lack of understanding what the user needs to be able to do with the technology. The coding techniques introduced in this chapter can be applied to analyze data collected from usability testing methods described in subsequent chapters, such as cognitive walkthroughs and think-alouds.

- *Chapter 7: Pre-design Studies.* This chapter describes the types of inquiry that should be used prior to beginning the design of a HIT product. The chapter focuses on formative testing, where the researcher is conducting user research and seeking to discover how target users will actually interact with the product they are designing and what contextual and subjective factors affect usability. The methods discussed in this chapter aim to under-stand the users for whom the HIT is being designed, what they intend to use it for, the types of interactions they may have with the product, and the context in which the HIT will be used. Both formal and informal methods will be discussed, including field observations, diary studies, focus groups, interviews, and surveys.

- *Chapter 8: Usability Inspection Methods.* This chapter describes more traditional formative usability testing methods, such as those that are conducted with experts only and those conducted with end-users. This chapter describes how to perform the various usability testing techniques that generally obtain qualitative data, such as think-aloud usability testing, including how many representative users are needed, how to recruit human subjects, developing real-life testing scenarios, and in what con-text to perform the study.

- *Chapter 9: Quantitative Usability Testing Methods and Metrics.* This chapter describes how to perform various usability tests that generally obtain quantitative data and how this data can be attributed to usability problems, such as frequency of task completion success versus failure and eye-tracking data. This chapter covers summative methods that can be completed after a HIT has been implemented and is already being used.

- *Chapter 10: Post-study Surveys and Retrospective Questionnaires.* This chapter introduces several standardized scales that measure UX or some aspect of it, including the popular and highly leveraged System Usability Scale (SUS). Several other common post-study usability scales are introduced, including the Post-study System Usability Questionnaire (PSSUQ), the Telemedicine Satisfaction and Usefulness Questionnaire (TSUQ), the Questionnaire for User Interface Satisfaction (QUIS), and the NASA-Task Load Index (NASA-TLX).
- *Chapter 11: Conclusion.* This concluding chapter summarizes the key takeaways of the text: how to develop research inquiries and select the best mixture of methods that will allow you to answer your research questions. It encourages readers to perform interdisciplinary, collaborative research and to mix methods, as well as to use the information to iteratively design usable HIT.

The chapters on methods begin with a description of the method and how usability is being evaluated or measured using the method. The type of data collected, evaluation apparatus or data collection instruments used, and data analysis techniques appropriate for the method, are discussed, followed by a few examples of studies that have used the methods in a usability study of HIT. Each method chapter ends with a recommendation on how the method is best combined with other usability evaluation methods. The methods are not explained in great detail, as discussion of each method could fill an entire book. Rather, this book is intended to provide a brief overview of the many usability evaluation methods that can be performed in conjunction with one another in a mixed-methods usability study of HIT to gain a better understanding of usability and be able to use the insight to design and deliver more usable HIT that improve the health of individuals.

WHAT IS NOT INCLUDED IN THIS BOOK

Given that there are numerous qualitative and quantitative methods to investigate, explore, illustrate, understand, measure, and test UX, not every possible method or use case can be explicated in this book. In addition, I encourage researchers and practitioners to modify methods and techniques in ways that support their investigation, study design, and available resources. I encourage researchers and practitioners to use different tools that support capturing relevant data and create novel data collection instruments where there is not one single instrument that already exists to be able to obtain the insight that one needs. Some UX methods and artifacts that are often used in the industry that are not discussed in this book, yet they are of no less importance in the full system design lifecycle. These include:

- data mining
- card sorting (and tree testing)
- market research
- competitive research
- action research
- user personal development
- customer/user journey mapping
- workflow analysis
- concept testing
- A/B testing
- PURE Method
- Clickstream Analysis.

A NOTE FROM THE AUTHOR

I was motivated to write this book following the completion of my dissertation study, which was a mixed-methods examination of telemedicine interfaces. I had to surf through a great deal of literature to understand what factors affected usability in the HCI of HIT and to learn how to design a study that could obtain the type of data I needed that would enable me to answer my research questions. I researched and took from literature in multiple disciplines: health and medical, technical communication, HCI, cognitive science, and more. This book aims to synthesize my research into an easy-to-read guide that helps researchers and practitioners design mixed-methods usability studies that will lead to the design and delivery of more usable HIT, which it is anticipated will lead to positive health outcomes.

2

Definitions: Usability, UX, and UCD

INTRODUCTION

This chapter provides an evolutionary history of usability and multiple definitions of usability, as well as the metrics against which usability has been tested. The four-step user-centered design (UCD) process will be detailed and alternative names for the UCD process will be discussed to demonstrate that UCD is an iterative process of working with real end-users to design and develop usable products.

USABILITY BY ANY OTHER NAME WOULD NOT BE AS COMPLEX

Usability, simply put, refers to how easy it is for an individual to use a product or technology to accomplish a particular task successfully. Yet usability is a complex and dynamic concept that has many definitions, which challenges practitioners and scholars to investigate and articulate the extent to which a product or technology is usable. The difficulty in studying usability stems from the many definitions that have been formulated and exist in the overlapping fields of human–computer interaction (HCI), user experience (UX), and technical communication (TC), as well as the various qualities of usability that are determined to be measurable. The variety of technologies and contexts for which usability can be investigated further complicates the ability to express usability and measure certain attributes, much less design rigorous and comprehensive usability studies. This chapter will begin with a survey of the commonly recognized definitions of usability, and the usability metrics and heuristics that evolved from the basic definition of usability. It will end with a description

DOI: 10.1201/9781003460886-2

of the four main user-centered design (UCD) steps to be performed in a full system design lifecycle.

International Organization of Standardization

ISO 9241-11

Arguably, the most recognized and frequently cited definition of usability is provided by the International Organization of Standardization (ISO). Presented in ISO 9241-11, usability is defined as "the extent to which a product can be used by specified users to achieve specified goals with effectiveness, efficiency, and satisfaction in a specified context of use" (ISO, 2018). Yen and Bakken (2012) summarize the ISO usability definition as "the ability of a product or application to be understood, learned, used, and aesthetically pleasing to the user within a specific context of use." Effectiveness refers to the accuracy and completeness with which a user is able to achieve their goals for users, and efficiency is the resources expended in relation to the effectiveness with which users achieve specified goals (ISO, 2018).

The ISO/IEC 9126:1991/2001 quality model classifies usability as one of six qualities of a technology: functionality, reliability, usability, efficiency, maintainability, and portability. Under the product quality model, usability consists of five attributes: understandability, learnability, operability, attractiveness, and usability compliance. The ISO offers a concrete description of each of these usability attributes—for instance, understandability is defined as the "capability of the software product to enable the user to understand whether the software is suitable and how it can be used for particular tasks and conditions of use" (ISO, 1991, 2001).

ISO/IEC 25010:2011

The definition of usability was further refined in 2017, when the ISO replaced the ISO/IEC 9126:1991 with the ISO/IEC 25010:2011 (ISO, 2017). According to the ISO/IEC 25010:2011, usability is the product of both the quality of use and the quality of the technology (ISO, 2017). *Usability is thus a product of both the user interaction and the design of the user interface.*

Extending on the previous ISO/IEC 9126:1991/2001, the usability of the interaction with a technology or product includes the following attributes: effectiveness, efficiency, satisfaction, freedom from risk, and context coverage (ISO, 2017). Also, according to the ISO/IEC 25010:2011 product quality model, the usability of the actual technology or product includes the following characteristics: functional suitability, reliability, performance efficiency, usability, security, compatibility, maintainability, and portability (ISO, 2017). Similarly, these eight characteristics are made more granular in the ISO/IEC 25010:2011, with each having its own defining characteristics (ISO, 2017).

Early Usability Criteria: Shackel

Shackel (1981) offers an initial and comprehensive definition of usability: the capability of a system to be easily and effectively used by a specified range of users, whom are given specified training and support, to fulfil a specified range of tasks, within a specified context. Shackel's (1981) broad definition emphasizes human users doing tasks in a specific context of use. Shackel (1981) considers usability to be something able to be measured by predetermined numerical values for each of the following criteria: effectiveness, learnability, flexibility, and attitude. These usability metrics are quantifiable requirements that can specified during the design of a system and evaluated to determine whether a system has sufficient usability. For instance, effectiveness is measured in terms of the speed in which tasks are accomplished by users; learnability can be quantified by determining an acceptable level of training and user support that a new user should maximumly require to be considered usable.

Shackel's (1981) conception of usability is important because it was the first to connect usability with the interaction between a user and the technology within a particular context. Shackel (1981) recognized that usability was impacted by human behavior and the design of the technology, as well as the context in which the interaction between the human and technology takes place. The relationship between these three aspects is important because they all affect usability and shape the user experience. A detailed explanation of usability determinants of HIT is provided in the next chapter.

Jacob Nielsen

Anyone who is interested in the design of technology, or is a practitioner or researcher in the fields of HCI, user experience, and/or usability engineering, is likely familiar with Jacob Nielsen. I consider Nielsen to be one of the godfathers of usability. Nielsen and colleagues began performing usability inspections using various methods and publishing about their methods and experiences in the late 1980s and early 1990s (Nielsen, 1994b, 1995; Nielsen & Mack, 1994).

Nielsen (1993a) specifies five usability attributes that are commonly used as metrics in usability studies. Nielsen (1993a) was certain to mention that usability is not one-dimensional, but generally consists of the following attributes:

- Learnability
- Efficiency
- Memorability
- Prevention of errors
- Satisfaction.

When specifically applied to HCI, Nielsen and Molich (1990) developed 10 usability heuristics that were later revised by Nielsen (1994b) to be leveraged as general principles for designing for usability:

1. Visibility of system status
2. Match between system and the real world
3. User control and freedom
4. Consistency and standards
5. Error prevention
6. Recognition rather than recall
7. Flexibility and efficiency of use
8. Aesthetic and minimalist design
9. Help users recognize, diagnose, and recover from errors
10. Help and documentation.

Don Norman

The other godfather of usability, Don Norman (2013), describes usability in terms of the affordances a technology offers users, but in concurrence with the ISO/IEC 25010:2011 (ISO, 2017), usability is described as both a quality of the user interaction and the design of the technology. Norman (2013, p. 11) states that "an affordance is a relationship between the properties of an object and the capabilities of the agent that determine just how the object could possibly be used." Norman's (2013) description expresses the difficulty with measuring usability, given that each unique individual may interact with a technology and be able to perceive or detect many affordances or none at all. In addition, different contexts in which a product is used also impact usability and the affordances that users are able to discover during the interaction. "The presence of an affordance is jointly determined by the qualities of the object and the abilities of the agent that is interacting" (Norman, 2013, p. 11).

Like Nielsen (1994b), Norman (2013) provides not a definition of usability, but rather certain criteria or properties exhibited by a product that has "good" usability:

- Retrievability
- Learnability
- Efficiency of use
- Ease of use (at first encounter)
- Aesthetics.

Norman (2013) suggests that usability is not a construct that is generally noticed until you test the product or system with representative users doing typical tasks they would likely perform when interacting with the product. In this context, good or poor usability is able to be revealed. Therefore, Norman's (2013) usability criteria can act like goals or heuristics by which to measure for or predict usability.

Designing User Interfaces for Usability

In, *Designing the User Interface*, Shneiderman and Plaisant (2010) favor a practical approach to usability and developed usability metrics that could be evaluated against:

1. Time to learn
2. Speed of performance
3. Rate of errors by users
4. Retention over time
5. Subjective satisfaction

Shneiderman and Plaisant's (2010) usability metrics collect mostly quantitative data that illustrate trends toward good or poor usability, with the exception of subjective satisfaction, which collects and analyzes qualitative data.

Preece and the Critical Issue of Safety

In 1994, Preece et al. (1994) added the attribute of safety to the standard definition of usability due to the large aim to design and delivery usable

HIT that are effective but, more importantly—because HIT involves human lives and health—also safe to use (Borycki & Kushniruk, 2005). Preece et al. (2002) define usability as a measure of how efficient, effective, enjoyable, and safe a computer system is to use. They consider safety to be a critical component of usability, thereby adding "safety" to Nielsen's five characteristics of usability:

- Effectiveness
- Efficiency
- Safety
- Utility
- Learnability
- Memorability (Preece et al., 2002).

The Implications of Technical Communication

Dumas and Redish (1999, p. 4) consider usability to mean "that the people who use the product can do so quickly and easily to accomplish their own tasks." Both Dumas and Redish, as technical communicators, emphasize four key user-focused principles of usability:

1. Usability means focusing on users.
2. People use products to be productive.
3. Users are busy people trying to accomplish tasks.
4. Users decide when a product is ready to use.

THE EVOLUTION OF USABILITY

The definition of usability has evolved and there is still no fixed set of usability attributes (Bruno & al-Qaimari, 2004; Nassar, 2012); however, all usability definitions, qualities, and criteria have a common thread: usability is determined by the user, the context of use, and the design of the product or interface with which the user interacts. *Usability is a product of individual or subjective factors as well as contextual or external factors.* Understanding that usability is dynamic empowers designers and practitioners to design usability studies that can evaluate usability using the most effective and feasible approach that will enable them to gain the knowledge and insight they need to iteratively design for usability. Whatever definition or metrics you use to test usability, it is critical that you have knowledge of the target users, the tasks they will perform with the technology, and the context within which they will interact with the technology. Having knowledge of these key variables will enable you to design a rigorous usability study.

Why User-Friendliness is Arbitrary

You might note that the term "user-friendliness" has not been mentioned in any definition of usability. Considering that usability is a product of the individual user and the interaction any one user has with technology, user-friendliness becomes a very arbitrary unit of measurement. Each individual user will have a different interaction with a technology based on numerous subjective characteristics, such as their level of knowledge of the technology, their physical capabilities, and their mood, in addition to the various contexts of use within which each interaction could take place. Therefore, operationally defining user-friendliness becomes problematic, and thus several practitioners in the HCI discipline have banned the term from their vocabulary (Nielsen, 1993a; Norman & Draper, 1986).

USEFULNESS

The discrimination between usability and usefulness is expressed by many HCI practitioners and in usability scholarship (Gangwar et al., 2014; Schillewaert et al., 2005; Yen et al., 2017); usefulness is argued to be as essential to the user experience as usability is (Mirel, 2004). Zhang and Walji (2011, p.1056) describe usability as "how useful, usable, and satisfying a system is for the intended users to accomplish goals" and refer to "usefulness" as how well a system supports the ability of the users to accomplish their goals for use. A product can have a sufficient level of usability, but if it is not useful, or serves "no recognizable purpose" (Grudin, 1992, p. 209), it will not be utilized or receive widespread adoption. Like usability, Mirel (2004) considers usefulness a value of the user experience. Usefulness is not whether an application or system is easy to use, but whether the system successfully makes it easier for a user to perform their job or do their work (Mirel, 2004). Mirel (2004) discriminates between usability and usefulness, but argues that neither design objective is less important to the user experience. Usefulness characterizes the tasks and functions a user needs to be able to accomplish to support their work; usability characterizes the ease of use, accessibility, navigation, and learnability of a product (Mirel, 2004).

The technology acceptance model (TAM) of information systems proposes that users' decision to accept and use a new technology depends on two integrating variables: perceived usefulness and perceived ease of use. The emphasis on a user's perception implies that user acceptance of a technology is partially a subjective opinion or determination, similar to how usability is affected by both subjective and contextual factors associated with the interaction between the human and technology. Upon initial or continued use of a technology, users innately perform a cost-benefit analysis of their interaction with the technology. If the perceived potential benefits, such as increased work productivity or efficiency, do not outweigh the difficulty in using the system, users will simply not utilize a system (Davis, 1989). Davis (1989) suggests that two key variables determine system use, and that these can be measured and have predictive value for usage behavior:

- *Perceived usefulness* is "the degree to which a person believes that using a particular system would enhance their job performance" (Davis, 1989, p. 320).
- *Perceived ease of use* is "the degree to which a person believes that using a system would be free of effort" (Davis, 1989, p. 320).

Thus, usefulness is a key variable that is directly correlated to usage behavior and user acceptance (Davis, 1989). If the potential of HIT to improve healthcare access and delivery, disease treatment, clinical diagnoses and decision-making, patient education, and all the other posited affordances of HIT is to be reached (Ammenwerth, 2015; Kellermann & Jones, 2013), HIT must be usable and useful for the intended users. Buchanan and Salako (2009) identified key attributes and associated measures of system usefulness as relevance, reliability, and currency.

Therefore, when designing HIT, not only usability but usefulness must be considered. HIT must convey to users—through its design and functionality—that they will be successful in accomplishing the tasks they expect to achieve by using the technology. Self-efficacy is another important factor that influences different users' behaviors and decisions. Self-efficacy is an individual's conviction that they will be successful at performing a task (Bandura, 1982). A HIT that is easy to use can increase a user's self-efficacy, and thus the likelihood that they will use the system. Research demonstrates that perceived ease of use influences perceived usefulness and ultimately affects the acceptance and adoption of HIT (Tang et al., 2019).

Usefulness versus Utility

Nielsen (2012) identifies "usefulness" and "utility" as two separate entities, but I consider them one in the same; usefulness and utility both have to do with the function of the technology or product and the purpose it serves and its ability to meet the needs of users. Overall, research on technology acceptance, and user behavior and decision-making processes, distinguishes and emphasizes the role of both subjective and objective factors in determining usability, and inevitably whether users will utilize a technology that is designed and delivered to them.

USER EXPERIENCE

Increasingly, usability is tied to user experience (UX) due to the emphasis on user satisfaction and the need to understand the user's subjective perception of their interaction with the product (ISO, 2018; Monkman & Griffith, 2021).

What is UX? UX is "a person's perceptions and responses that result from the use or anticipated use of a product, system or service" (ISO, 2018). Norman and Nielsen (n.d.) describe UX as encompassing "all aspects of the end-user's interaction with the company, its services, and its products." Usability is a fundamental component of UX, but UX extends beyond usability to include all the multiple touchpoints that a person has with technology and humans throughout their initial and ongoing use of a technology, including their perceptions and the responses that are engendered from their experience. Think of UX as a composite of every transaction a user has with a company, which likely includes a network of interactions between humans and technology.

UX of HIT Example

DTC telemedicine is a modern healthcare delivery system that utilizes a variety of digital technology, multimedia, and interactive communication platforms to facilitate diagnosis, consultation, treatment, the transfer of medical data, education, and communication between multiple stakeholders (i.e. physician to physician; physician to patient; caretakers, nurses, etc.) (Bashshur, 1995). Direct-to-consumer (DTC) telemedicine is the delivery of healthcare for non-emergency conditions to the general public via a live video chat using a webcam or smartphone, or simply via a telephone call with a physician (Bollmeier et al., 2020; Uscher-Pines et al, 2016). In the United States, DTC telemedicine is commonly known as virtual physician visits or remote doctor visits, and is provided by large telemedicine providers, such as Amwell, MD Live, MeMD, and Teladoc (Resneck et al., 2016; Uscher-Pines & Mehrotra, 2014).

Telemedicine providers, like other healthcare providers and businesses, market their service through their consumer-facing website. An individual's knowledge of telemedicine and how to use a telemedicine service is obtained from the individual's initial access to and interaction with the telemedicine provider website. A user's first interaction with the website is a part of the UX of the telemedicine service. As users interact with the telemedicine website, they may need to read and comprehend information and perform certain actions, such as registering to be a patient and downloading an application, in order to be able to schedule a virtual consultation with a telemedicine doctor. All these interactions are a part of the UX. When a patient performs the virtual doctor visit and is able to receive treatment for their health condition, such as getting prescription medications automatically sent to their pharmacy, these interactions with the doctor and pharmacy are a part of the UX. Lastly, any follow-up communications from the telemedicine service, such as emails to the patient or a follow-up call from the physician, are a part of the UX and would likely lead to a patient's positive perception of the telemedicine service. All the interactions the user has with the telemedicine company, from their initial interaction with the telemedicine website, to their interaction with the remote communication platform, to their interaction with the physician, and to their interaction with any follow-up communications, must all have a sufficient level of usability to shape the UX.

UX designers and marketing professionals might refer to UX as the consumer journey because it illustrates the types of tasks and actions a human may need to perform and the interactions a human may encounter on their technology use journey. Considering that usability is determined by both the subjective and contextual factors involved in an individual's unique interaction with technology, usability shapes UX.

HUMAN–COMPUTER INTERACTION

Usability is often tied to the field of human–computer interaction (HCI) because most of human work and daily life is reliant on computers and the use of digital technology, which is the focus of this book. The modern healthcare system leverages many interoperable and disparate forms of technology and systems to improve healthcare delivery, patient treatment, and health maintenance.

Increasingly, people use HIT, such as health information websites, mobile health applications, and Fitbits, to track, maintain, and gain knowledge about their health. Like technical communication, HCI is an interdisciplinary field and, like usability, HCI has no general and unified theory. However, HCI has identical threads with technical communication, which connect the three foci of usability: the people, the computers, and the tasks that are performed (Dix et al. 2004). The conditions that must be met for product succuss are usefulness, usable, and used. The last condition—used—which Dix et al. (2004) describe as a product that makes people want to use it because it is motivating and attractive, ties more to the user experience (Dix et al., 2004), and emphasizes the significance of user satisfaction, enjoyment, and pleasure during the experience of interacting with a technology.

Usability Engineering

The field concerned with building usability into a product is called "usability engineering" (Dumas & Redish, 1999; Whiteside et al., 1988). Usability engineering is not so much a discipline as a set of methods and procedures that can be performed during the design and development of a technology in order to ensure that the final end product is usable. In usability engineering, insight about usability is the central focus in the initial stages of the full system design lifecycle, which is often not the case in most development contexts (Mirel, 2004). Usability is most often evaluated after a product has already been finalized and delivered to target users. When usability is considered a "downstream process" (Mirel, 2004, p. xxxii), software teams do not have the ability to apply the insights obtained about usability to their decisions about the design and functionality of the product. Usability engineering considers usability crucial for determining front-end, high-level requirements for a system, and throughout the entire full system design lifecycle (Mirel, 2004).

User-centered design (UCD) (described next) is a process that aims to design and develop usable products by involving end-users in the design and development stages of a product and performing usability tests that obtain insight, which can facilitate iterative design changes that improve usability. UCD, as such, can be considered a specific methodology performed by usability engineers and technical communicators aimed to design and deliver usable products. Usability engineering, of course, includes many other methods to obtain knowledge of the intended audience, the tasks they need to be able to perform, and the context of use, as well as testing methods that will be discussed in this book, but often UCD includes the use of these methods throughout the full system design lifecycle.

Usability engineering positions usability and usefulness as key concerns early in the design and development phases of the full system design lifecycle (Mirel, 2004). Because UCD is considered an approach to designing usable products, it falls under the technical communication and HCI umbrella because its primary purpose is to design usable products and its approach to doing so is working with real-end users throughout the full system design lifecycle.

USER-CENTERED DESIGN (UCD)

When you are designing HIT to be usable, how do you know how to design a system so it meets the needs, wants, and expectations of the target users? In addition, how are you able to understand how the various health literacy levels and contextual factors affect the usability of target users' interaction with HIT? You ask them! This is a simple way of describing the method of UCD. UCD is an iterative design method, whereby you include end-users in the design and development stages of a technology in order to discover more about them, gain a better understanding of their needs and how they will actually use the technology, and obtain feedback that can be used to inform design changes in the technology to improve usability.

As early as the 1970s, technical communication's implications for the design and delivery of usable products originated from the critical focus on delivering technical and complex communications to intended users and ensuring they were able to read, comprehend, and perform tasks successfully using technical documents (Redish, 2010). Technical communicators ensured their products were usable by performing a series of steps, including user research and usability testing of their products with a sample of users who best represented the population of target users. With its roots in technical communication, which is an interdisciplinary field in itself (Redish, 2010; St.Amant, 2020), UCD is a practical approach to designing and developing usable systems by involving end-users in the design and development stages. UCD was founded on three key principles outlined by Gould and Lewis (1985):

1. An early focus on users and the tasks they perform. This step is performed to access users' cognitive, behavioral, anthropometric, and attitudinal characteristics.

2. An empirical measurement using simulations and prototypes to observe users executing their real work and be able to record and analyze their reactions.
3. The performance of iterative design. Iterative design consists of the continuous testing with end-users and using their feedback to make design changes that improve the usability of the product.

Gould et al. (1985) advocate that users must be a part of the development of a system because they are the people to whom the product is intended to be for whom it will be used to achieve anticipated outcomes. UCD leverages the theoretical knowledge and expertise of several disciplines: cognitive science, psychology, computer science, sociology, linguistics, anthropology, and more (Dix et al., 2004; Mayhew, 1999; Norman et al., 1986), and thus borrows from interdisciplinary research and design techniques to study users and design usable products. Usability has been a critical focus by the U.S. Office of the National Coordinator for Health Information Technology (ONC) since mandating that HIT technology vendors certify that EHRs are designed and implemented according to certain criteria specified in the Code of Federal Regulations §170.314(g)(3) (2010). EHR developers are required to demonstrate that UCD has been adopted to design the HIT and that various usability testing and safety evaluations have been completed (Buchanan et al., 2014).

Four-Step Process

To expand on Gould et al.'s (1985) principles for designing usable products, UCD has developed into a full system design process consisting of four steps that are repeated to create an iterative design lifecycle (see Figure 2.1):

1. *Perform user research/audience analysis (discovery).* At the start of a new project, you will first want to get to know your audience—the intended users of the technology you are designing. This involves collaborating with individuals who best represent the end-users of the product. You identify their needs, the primary context in which they will use the technology, and other subjective and contextual factors that may impact usability, such as their literacy levels, physical abilities, and social and cultural practices.
2. *Specify system requirements (explore).* This step requires that you gain a sense of what the users must be able to accomplish by using the technology. Essentially, you answer the questions: What do the users need to be able to do when interacting with the technology? And what goals do

Perform user research / Audience Analysis

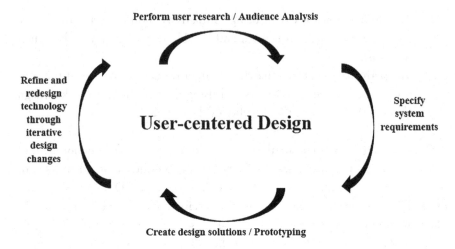

User-centered Design

Refine and redesign technology through iterative design changes

Specify system requirements

Create design solutions / Prototyping

FIGURE 2.1
User-centered design (UCD) illustrated as a four-step process formulating the iterative, full-system design lifecycle.

they need to achieve from using the technology? This step is often when you develop a list of specifications for the technology you are developing, such as a list of functions it must be capable of. The user goals you list may also become metrics for which you can test later in the design product to demonstrate the product is successful.

3. *Create design solutions/prototyping (design).* In this stage, once you understand who the technology is for and what they need to be able to accomplish by using the technology, you design the technology using sketches of initial design concepts, low- or high-fidelity prototypes or functional model of the technology, then you test with real end-users. In this stage, you evaluate usability and identify usability problems, as well as gain subjective user feedback of their interaction with the product. The data and insight you gain from usability testing is used in the final stage of UCD.

4. *Refine and redesign technology through iterative design changes (test).* In this step, you use the user feedback and insight you gained from the usability evaluations you performed in step three to make changes in the design of the technology in ways that will improve usability. For instance, if during usability testing you discovered that several of your user participants did not understand the function of a button because the icon used did not match their expectations, in this step you would be able to implement an icon that better represented the function to ensure users were able to interpret it correctly. Steps 3 and 4 are repeated so you can make iterative

design changes or incremental refinements in the technology until you reach a final product that has optimal usability or meets the requirements for product success that have been predetermined by you, your design team, and likely the business or company for which you are creating the technology.

Three Times a Charm

Generally, at least three design iterations are required to discover and resolve most of the major design flaws that create usability problems (Nielsen, 1993b). Certain usability parameters may be focused on during one design iteration and others may be overlooked until the second design iteration. Additionally, once changing a system, you can inherently create new usability problems for users so continuous usability evaluations and testing ensure that the final product will enable users to accomplish their goals easily, effectively, and efficiently. However, after about three iterations, a point is reached where the median improvement per iteration will drop and further usability testing may not be cost-effective or feasible.

OTHER TERMS FOR UCD

UCD has been widely adopted by the HCI and UX communities, and has been reclaimed under different names, but the focus is always on the user—the human for whom the technology is intended—and the end-goal is always to design and deliver usable products.

- *User-centered system design* is the term used by Norman et al. (1986). UCD is just a shorter form of user-centered system design. Norman et al. (1986, p. 2) state that, "The emphasis is on people, rather than technology, although the powers and limits of contemporary machines are considered in order to know how to take that next step from today's limited machines toward more user-centered ones." Throughout their text, Norman et al. (1986) encourage designers and researchers to be flexible and leverage interdisciplinary knowledge to approach designing technology for usability. They emphasize the social and organizational aspects of HCI within a specific context that impacts usability, and stress that there is no one-size-fits-all approach to design or working with end-users because every HCI is unique.

- *Usability engineering* (UE) (Dumas et al., 1999) is not necessarily a replacement term for UCD, but it parallels the iterative, full-system design lifecycle that UCD prescribes. "Usability engineering stars with identifying users, analyzing tasks, and setting usability specifications, moves on through developing and testing prototypes, and continues through interactive cycles of development and testing" (Dumas et al., 1999, p. 9). Dumas et al. (1999, p. 5) remind us of Gould et al.'s (1985) principles for designing usable products and parallel UCD with usability engineering: "To develop a usable product, you have to know, understand, and work with people who represent the actual or potential users of the product. No one can substitute for them." Early usability engineering handbooks similarly describe usability engineering as a "discipline that provides structured methods for achieving usability in user interface design during product development" (Mayhew, 1999, p. 2) and that reinforces the interdisciplinary perspectives required to successfully achieve usability in product design and development (Mayhew, 1999).
- *Human-centered design (HCD)* is increasingly replacing UCD as the name describing the philosophy that seeks to place the user at the center of the design process (Harte et al., 2017; ISO, 2019). HCD also underscores the human factors or cognitive-socio-technical-cultural aspects that impact usability (Carroll, 1997). HCD requires empathy to be able to understand how and why humans do certain things when they interact with technology in order to be able to design for usability. Many health informatics scholars have embraced this term, as it "focuses on using multidisciplinary teams and on an iterative design process, in which feedback from users is a critical source of information" (Demiris et al., 2010; Kushniruk et al., 1997, 2004, 2008).
- *Interaction design* is Mirel's (2004) solution to the neglect of usability and usefulness in most software development contexts. Usefulness is the primary aim of interaction design, and usefulness (like usability is to UCD) is considered right at the beginning of the full system design lifecycle (Beck, 2000). Interaction design includes obtaining contextually derived requirements, such as "how people desire to use a product for work-related goals, why, and with what patterns of behavior" (Mirel, 2004, p. xxxiii) in order to design a product that is easy to use and useful to the those who are going to use it in the context of their work.
- *User-interface design* is the dynamic process that Shneiderman et al. (2010) describe as using tools, design techniques, and specific methods to support design consistency, universal usability, and evolutionary refinement.

User-interface design requires planning, sensitivity to users' needs, analysis of requirements, usability testing, and remaining within budgets and deliverable deadlines. "Great designers are deeply committed to serving the users, which strengthen their resolve when they face difficult choices, time pressures, and tight budgets" (Shneiderman et al., 2010, p. 13). As suggested by Shneiderman et al. (2010), the user-interface design process requires interaction with end-users early in the design phase, is iterative, and leverages user feedback to make incremental refinements in the design to improve usability.

• *Participatory design* (Spinuzzi, 2005) emphasizes the methodological function of UCD to conduct rigorous user research through user involvement. Spinuzzi (2005, p. 164) states that, "The approach is just as much about design—producing artifacts, systems, work organizations, and practical or tacit knowledge—as it is about research." Spinuzzi (2005) suggests that various research methods are used to iteratively construct the emerging design, which is resultantly, co-designed by the end-users who participate in the participatory design process. The iterative co-design process draws on various research methods, including ethnographic observations, interviews, analysis of artifacts, and protocol analysis, among others, to systematically collect data that can be analyzed and offer insights that can be used to build usable products.

There are many alternative names for UCD; however, I consider them all to be the same because the primary purpose of UCD is to design and deliver usable products, and the approach to doing so involves working with real-end users, performing various user research and testing methods, and making iterative design changes to improve the usability of the product until an agreed upon minimal number of usability problems exist or optimal usability has been achieved.

SUMMARY

The main premise of this chapter is to demonstrate that there are various similar usability definitions and criteria for measuring usability, which are associated with a range of usability qualities. Furthermore, usability is affected by both the individual characteristics of the user, aspects related to the context in which the user interacts with the product, the tasks the user sets out to accomplish during their interactions, and the design of the user interface in which the interaction between a user and the technology takes place. Given the complexity in the understanding of usability, the various ways in which usability can be measured, and the individual and contextual factors that affect usability, usability is a construct that is best suited for mixed-methods studies that involve the use of many different and uniquely designed methods.

3

Audience Analysis and Usability Determinants

INTRODUCTION

Given that usability is an intricate, context-specific, dynamic, and multidimensional phenomenon, this chapter attempts to identify, classify, and describe the multidimensional factors that affect usability. In doing so, researchers and practitioners gain a comprehensive and holistic perspective of usability and the many ways in which it can be observed, evaluated, and measured, thereby underscoring the notion that usability is a phenomenon that cannot be investigated using a single method. The chapter ends with a brief discussion of formative and summative usability testing and where they fit into the full system design lifecycle.

KNOW YOUR AUDIENCE

A usability evaluation addresses the interaction between the user and a system (Nielsen, 1993a); therefore, one of the first steps in designing a usability study, and similarly in UCD, is to understand your audience—the intended user of the technology you are designing and evaluating. The audience, or user population, consists of the individuals who will actually use or interact with the HIT to be able to do something, such as perform a health-related behavior, or be able to achieve a specific health-related goal or outcome as a result of interacting with the HIT.

Within the fields of HCI, usability/UX, and technical communication, the term "user" is commonly used to refer to the human group or population who are the intended users of the document or system you are designing. "User" may sometimes be prefixed with the terms "target" or "end-" to reinforce the idea that the technology should be designed in such a way as to facilitate and optimize the interaction between the human who the technology is supposed to help. "User" is often used interchangeably with the terms "audience" and "population" if you are discussing technology design and delivery, or "subject," "participant," or "respondent" if you are discussing a usability study that includes the participation of end-users. In either case, it is important that you understand the target users of the HIT you are going to test.

Conducting an audience analysis is the first step to getting to know the users for whom the HIT is being designed. Users of HIT include a number of diverse stakeholders: clinicians, nurses, administrators, caregivers, patients, health insurers, and so on. "Stakeholders" refers to any individuals who interact with the HIT in any context; those who have a "stake" in the success of the technology, which is to say they are relying on the technology to help them achieve a specified goal. The importance of identifying and understanding target users of the technology being investigated arises from the definition of usability—the extent to which a product or technology can be used by a specified user to achieve specified goals in a particular context of use (ISO, 2018). Identifying your intended user or target audience allows you to better understand the multi-dimensional factors that affect the usability of that particular user's interaction with the technology under investigation.

INDIVIDUAL/SUBJECTIVE AND CONTEXTUAL/ EXTERNAL DETERMINANTS OF USABILITY

What are the multidimensional factors that affect the usability of HIT? Recalling that usability is affected by the interaction between the user and the technology implies that there are human factors influencing usability and user interface design aspects that influence usability. The multidimensional factors that affect usability can be differentiated as individual or subjective usability determinants and contextual or external usability determinants. Figure 3.1 illustrates the individual and contextual aspects that can affect a user within a specified context of use.

Individual or subjective factors that affect usability include social, cognitive, physical, and cultural factors, as well as individuals' unique health situations (Albers, 2003, Carliner, 2000; Goldberg et al., 2011). A contextual or external factor that affects usability is the physical environment in which users access HIT

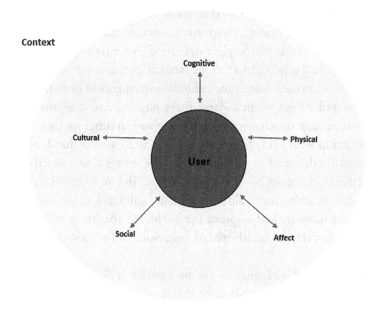

FIGURE 3.1

A multidimensional audience analysis includes a comprehensive understanding of the cognitive, physical, affect, social, and cultural factors that impact a user's interaction with HIT within a specific context of use.

(St.Amant, 2017). Additionally, the health information needs of users, which vary according to the health situation and context of use, can also be considered a contextual determinant of usability as they help to establish functionality requirements of a HIT (Kushniruk et al, 2008; Pang et al., 2016; Zhang et al., 2011). The individual and contextual factors that affect usability can further be classified as cognitive, physical, social, affect, and cultural factors that interconnect to affect usability within a context of use. As such, these classifications are not mutually exclusive. For instance, the physical characteristics of an individual, such as their vision and ability to perceive user interface elements, such as buttons, menu options, and text (Punchoojit & Hongwarittorrn, 2017), can be classified as individual usability determinants because these physical capabilities are highly unique to the individual. Yet physical attributes of a user's environment, such as the geographic location, the presence of other people, time available to perform a task, and the availability of certain medical instruments (Rizvi et al., 2017), certainly all affect usability, and are considered contextual variables. Furthermore, St.Amant (2021) describes that an individual's physical environment is perceived through a cognitive script (Schank & Abelson, 1977;

Tomkins, 1987), which is then used to guide the actions and behaviors a user performs in that environment. A cognitive script originates from an individual's repeated experience in a specific place over time. For instance, when entering a clinic, an individual might expect to see medical instruments and a doctor and expect the doctor to use some of the medical instruments to perform a physical examination and collect medical data. These physical and cognitive attributes are intertwined and simultaneously influence one another as they shape the user's interaction with HIT. St.Amant (2017, 2018) asserts that health information must be designed using content (words, images, user interface elements) that match the target user's cognitive script. The more an HIT can match a user's cognitive script for health-related and healthcare situations, the more it will increase usability and improve the likelihood that users will accept and use the HIT to perform health-related behaviors and achieve positive health outcomes.

The objective of this chapter is not to separate individual and contextual determinants of usability or advocate that one has greater influence on the user experience with HIT than the other, but rather to call attention to the multidimensions of a HCI with HITs that affect usability, which allows for practitioners to perform more comprehensive and complete audience analyses and researchers to be more precise when attempting to measure one or more variables that influence usability.

Kairos, or the opportune moment in terms of timing and circumstances (Aristotle, 1991) for users to interact with HIT is another important consideration that affects usability. In understanding usability, *kairos* means knowing the right time when, or right situation in which, users would most likely need access to HIT and therefore be more motivated and likely to utilize it. *Kairos* may also influence a user when participating in usability testing. Thus, *kairos* must be addressed when evaluating for usability, as well as when designing usability studies, as it is linked to both individual and contextual usability determinants.

Individual and contextual usability determinants are intertwined and dynamic, and thus carry more or less weight during different times of the user interaction with technology. For example, under conditions that require a rapid response, such as in the Emergency Department (ED), clinicians may use more initiative-based decisions and require a clinical decision support system (CDSS) that allows for quick patient assessment and little documentation (Sheehan et al., 2013). The context of the ED requires that clinicians be able to interact with an CDSS and be able to cognitively process information accurately and quickly; therefore, the contextual factors may affect usability more than the individual factors do. In contrast, individual factors, such as a patient's limited health literacy, affect their ability to enter correct search terms in order to retrieve the specific online health information for which they are looking (Birru et al., 2004). In this case, individual usability determinants are more influential than contextual usability determinants. Yet the design of the user interface shapes the user interaction with HIT, and the way the information is displayed, navigational elements, and functionality can all promote or impede usability (Johnson et al., 2005). Figure 3.2 illustrates just a sample of the various multidimensional aspects of an individual, which vary according to the context of use.

The multidimensional and often changing individual characteristics and contexts in which an individual interacts with HIT must be taken into consideration when designing HIT and during the full system development lifestyle—for instance, when designing usability studies. Although an unlimited number of factors may affect a user when interacting with HIT because every individual is unique, as is every health situation, from a review and analysis of the scientific literature, I will next present the most critical factors known to impact the usability of HIT.

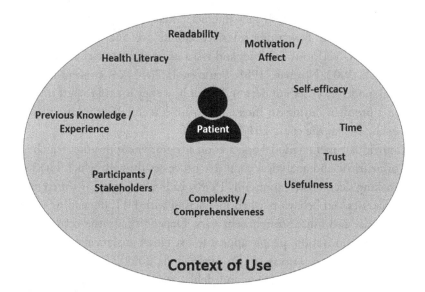

FIGURE 3.2
Various multidimensional aspects of an individual that affect usability within a specific context of use include motivation/affect, self-efficacy, health literacy, and previous experience/ knowledge can be considered individual usability determinants. Readability, time, complexity/ comprehensiveness, participants/stakeholders, and usefulness can be considered contextual usability determinants.

Individual/Subjective Determinants of Usability

Individual or subjective determinants of usability include aspects such as how a human processes information or how much they know about a subject. These characteristics are highly unique to every individual, but are also affected by environmental factors, such as how much time they have to perform a particular task (Damman et al., 2009) or whether they have others available to help them understand complex information (Demiris et al., 2010). Individual usability determinants are affected by contextual usability determinants and vice versa because usability cannot be detached from the context of use. However, in order to present the most significant factors that affect the usability of HIT, they will be classified as aspects that are mostly an individual or subjective characteristic and those that mostly stem from the environment or one's context of use.

Cognitive Model and the Continuum

Norman (1988) argues that individuals form mental models of how to behave and perform actions in the world, which is the integration of previous experience and knowledge, cultural conventions, and how they interpret the information and interfaces with which they interact. There is a gap between designers' conceptual models of how a user interface should look and function, and how the user actually performs activities and tasks using the interface to reach goals (Kinzie et al., 2002; Norman, 1988; Peute et al., 2015a). A conceptual model, or mental model, is a user's understanding of how they intend to perform a task or solve a problem during an interaction with a technology (Norman, 1988; Peute et al., 2015a; Xie et al., 2017).

An individual's mental model operates on a cognitive continuum, which is the series of heuristic and analytical cognitive processes through which one moves when making decisions (Hammond, 1998). Individuals employ different cognitive processes and behaviors when interacting with HIT, depending on their mental model and innate search behaviors. Depending on the context of use and the user's motivation, people appear to use either analytical or experiential modes of information processing (Damman et al., 2009). The analytical mode of information processing is slow and deliberate. Users are highly motivated to search for health information and use logic and reasoning in order to determine if the information they find is of sufficient quality and likely to be useful (Damman et al., 2009; Sillence et al., 2006). Users employ a more superficial, quick judgement of health information based on heuristics and affect when using the experimental mode of information processing (Damman et al., 2009;

Sillence et al., 2006). Users might employ the experimental mode of information processing if they are not highly motivated or have an urgent need to find information quickly. Other scholars call these routes of information processing the central route or the peripheral route (Freeman & Spyridakis, 2004). The central route is used when an individual is making a conscious cognitive effort to process information, and the peripheral route is activated when users use cues to make quick judgments without having to employ much cognitive effort (Freeman et al., 2004).

Therefore, understanding a user's mental model of how they expect to interact with a HIT is essential to being able to design for usability. Understanding a user's cognitive model and continuum is equally as important when developing the artificial scenarios or tasks that users perform during usability testing. The more you can match a user's mental model, the more realistic you can be in designing a high-fidelity, quality study because users are more likely to perform as they would in a real-life situation.

Previous Knowledge and Experience

A well-known contributing factor to usability is an individual's previous knowledge of or experience with using a product or technology (Albers, 2003; Carroll & McKendree, 1986; Johnson et al., 2005). When interpreting symptoms provided by online health information websites, most individuals rely on matching symptoms with their existing medical knowledge or previous medical experiences (Luger et al., 2014). For instance, studies show that medical experts rely heavily on their previous knowledge—often in the form of mental schemas—and existing data to produce rapid, correct diagnoses, whereas novices use backward reasoning by first formulating a hypothesis then using data to make a diagnosis, which can result in incorrect diagnoses (Leprohon & Patel, 1995; Patel & Groen, 1986). However, individuals are not well equipped to predict their own health information needs, especially when experiencing a health crisis or an urgent health situation (Hibbard et al., 1997). Furthermore, research suggests that users are unable to recognize their own health information needs—or, if they do recognize their health information needs, they do not demand or access essential health information that may help them make appropriate decisions about their health, even if it is available (Alzougool et al., 2008). For example, individuals may recognize that they have a need for health information regarding treatment options for their disease, yet feel anxious and frightened about their health situation, so may refuse to access health information that is available online.

Users' health information needs, both recognized and unrecognized, change depending on the context in which they act on the health information, which is dynamic, as well as on the basis of individuals' willingness to act on the information (Alzougool et al., 2008). For instance, individuals may not demand health information regarding how to treat an illness until they become ill and require the health information. In another context of use, individuals may be unwilling to access essential health information or choose to ignore available health information because they believe it will make them anxious or worried, such as if an individual is going to have surgery and does not access online health information regarding post-surgical care. There is another group of health information users described as the "ignored group," comprising those individuals with "unrecognized, undemanded information needs" (Alzougool et al., 2008). Alzougool et al. (2008) refer to the "ignored group" as individuals who neither recognize their need for essential health information nor have the ability to act on it as a result of their context of use. It is often particularly challenging to meet the health information needs of the "ignored group," as it requires being able to predict their health information needs and deliver health information in multiple, easily accessible and recognizable ways because individuals may not accept some forms or types of available health information, such as that from a certain website or portal (Alzougool et al., 2008).

Alongside knowledge, Albers (2003) identifies two other primary components of an individual's mental model that shape the individual's interpretation, assimilation, and cognitive processing of dynamic or multimodal information: desire or need for detail and cognitive abilities. Designing usable information requires one to explore these multidimensions of individuals as they integrate and comprehend information (Albers, 2003). The detail dimension regards the level of detailed information a user desires or needs to achieve their goal for use (Albers, 2003) The cognitive dimension is concerned with users' ability to cognitive process information based on their own unique cognitive abilities, as different individuals have varying degrees of cognitive abilities (Albers, 2003). Understanding users' knowledge of a health subject, desire or need for detailed information, and cognitive processing abilities certainly has implications for designing HIS that are able to be used successfully by a target user population.

For instance, subjects interacting with health insurance information websites desired detailed information on the health plans, yet were also overwhelmed by the display of too much information on one page, which led to difficulty processing the information (Damman et al., 2009). Similarly, subjects interacting with a telemedicine website who aimed to set up a virtual doctor visit were hesitant to do so without having detailed information regarding the Teladoc credentials (Campbell & Monkman, 2021). A usability study of physicians' interactions with EHR discovered that the autopopulation feature simultaneously improved usability and hindered usability (Rizvi et al., 2017). The autopopulation function served as a catalytic agent to the note-writing process by automatically populating note fields, yet it also introduced usability problems by entering inaccurate, dated, or redundant information, causing the physicians to have to correct those fields and thus reducing efficiency (Rizvi et al., 2017). Likewise, clinicians' familiarity and experience with a health situation lead them to employ different decision-making strategies (Kushniruk, 2001). An experienced clinician may be able to make rapid diagnoses of a familiar medical condition, whereas a clinician whom has less medical expertise regarding a specific health condition may invoke analytical reasoning (Kushniruk, 2001).

Health Literacy

Health literacy, as defined by Weiss (2003, p. 4), is "an individual's ability to read, understand, and use healthcare information to make effective healthcare decisions and follow instructions for treatment." Several studies have demonstrated the importance of health literacy for users' ability to read and understand the health information they find, discern the quality of the information, and use the information appropriately to make informed decisions about their health and perform health behaviors (Bodie et al., 2008; Melonçon, 2016, 2017; Monkman et al., 2013b, 2015; Morony et al., 2017). Health literacy goes beyond just being able to read health information; it includes being able to access health information, comprehend it, and use it to perform health behaviors, and also to share in the decision-making process with their physician regarding treatment options (Artnak et al., 2011; Hsu et al., 2014; Melonçon, 2016; Melonçon, 2017; Monkman et al., 2013b). Health literacy encompasses listening and problem-solving, and is influenced by culture and societal factors (Ratzan & Parker, 2000). Most literature regarding health literacy tends to refer to eHealth literacy. Because so much health information is delivered and retrieved through the use of technology, health literacy often requires a sufficient level of computer literacy and internet access (Fox & Fallows, 2003; Hsu et al., 2014; Norman & Skinner, 2006). eHealth literacy involves a suitable knowledge of how to use health technologies in a particular context, and how to discriminate among online resources when accessing and using online health information (Agree et al., 2015). The mobile environment is another context of use that affects usability by affecting many of the other usability determinants, discussed next. When reading text on a mobile device, user comprehension may suffer or it may take an individual longer to read and comprehend information than when it is read on a desktop computer screen (Moran, 2016; Nielsen & Budiu, 2013). A mobile environment has been demonstrated to impact users' memory, focus, and navigation (Moran, 2016).

Health literacy and the usability of eHealth and other HIS are intricately connected. Users must be able to access health information from a variety of digital resources, such as websites and mobile health applications, comprehend the health information, and apply the information that is relevant to them to improve their health (Monkman et al., 2015). Likewise, health literacy levels have the potential to affect data quality, accuracy, and the usability of HIS— for instance, users may enter incorrect medical data into a PHR as a result of misunderstanding medical terminology (Monkman et al., 2013b).

Low health literacy is associated with a number of poor health criteria, such as more emergency care and hospitalizations, less use of preventative healthcare services, poor medication administration, and poor self-efficacy in managing health conditions (Berkman, et al., 2011). Agree et al. (2015) state that, "Low health literacy among older adults is compounded by the fact that older adults experience more chronic diseases, take more medications, and visit health care providers more often than younger adults." Health literacy has an intricate and intimate effect on the usability of telemedicine. Sarkar et al. (2010) identify low health literacy as a barrier to even being aware of alternative healthcare interventions, which may explain limited use among target populations. Ameliorating usability issues that are related to health literacy and context of use may result in an increased adoption and acceptance of telemedicine and may increase the positive health outcomes of users. These types of usability problems are able to be identified during usability tests, such as the think-aloud usability tests performed in my research.

Readability

Understanding that health literacy is an essential component if people are to successfully navigate and use complex health information to improve health outcomes, Wilson (2009) contends that reading level is one of the major determinants of health literacy and is a consideration when evaluating the usability of health information. Older adults, minority populations, and those in typically underserved geographic locations have statistically been shown to have poor health literacy (Berkman et al., 2011; Dewalt et al., 2004; Sandefer et al., 2015). Readability is the comprehension difficulty of text and is mathematically calculated. Wilson (2009) and the American Medical Association contends that health information should not be written at more than a sixth grade reading level (Weiss, 2003). If consumers are able to read, understand, and use eHealth tools effectively, it will increase the ability of these alternative health interventions to positively impact the health outcomes of those who use them—especially for racial minorities and those in typically under-served rural areas who have low health literacy and less access to healthcare (Dutta-Bergman, 2004; Krieger & Bassett, 1986; Kutner, et al., 2006; Uscher-Pines et al., 2014). It should be noted that readability does not equate with comprehension (a component of health literacy), but it does affect it (Dewalt et al., 2004; Nielsen, 2015; Nielsen & Budiu, 2013; Norman, 1988), which demonstrates the web of aspects of usability that must be considered when designing HIT for target audiences. Besides readability, which influences health literacy, one's context of use affects these usability factors as well. Nielsen Norman Group's readability studies show that even easy-to-read text becomes more difficult on mobile devices (Moran, 2016; Nielsen et al., 2013). The reading space is smaller, which reduces comprehension, and the need to scroll to read large passages of text degrades memory and takes more time.

Morony et al. (2017) regard readability as a proxy for or representative of usable health information. Birru et al. (2004) found that most of the online health information available was, on average, available at an eleventh grade reading level based on the Flesch-Kincaid Reading Scale. Overwhelmingly, the literature shows that health information providers are not cognizant of users' low health literacy levels, which is partially influenced by not delivering health information and patient education materials that are written at an appropriate reading level or that reflect the language and cultural values of the target user group (Wilson, 2009; Wilson et al., 2003). Health and medical professionals and clinicians are encouraged to perform readability assessments of the health information they provide to patients and recognize the impacts of health literacy and the effects it can have on individuals' health outcomes.

Motivation and Affect

Individuals' motivational and emotional state can impact their ability to understand and use health information or other HIT or appropriately in their context of use. Because health information is complex, humans have limited cognitive abilities to process and understand health information. Depending on the context of use and users' motivation, people appear to use either analytical or experiential modes of information processing (Damman et al., 2009). The analytical mode of information processing is slow and deliberate. Users are highly motivated to search for health information and use logic and reasoning in order to determine if the information they find is of sufficient quality and is going to be useful (Damman et al., 2009; Sillence et al., 2006). Users employ a more superficial, quick judgment of health information based on heuristics and affect when using the experimental mode of information processing (Damman et al., 2009; Sillence et al., 2006). Users might employ the experimental mode of information processing if they are not highly motivated or have an urgent need to find information quickly. Other scholars refer to these two different information processing routes as the "central route" and the "peripheral route" (Freeman et al., 2004). The central route is used when an individual is making a conscious cognitive effort to process information, and the peripheral route is activated when users use cues to make quick judgments without having to employ much cognitive effort (Freeman et al., 2004; Gigerenzer & Goldstein, 1996; Sillence et al., 2006). For instance, in highly urgent situations, nurses rely on simple rules to guide their decisions (Leprohon et al., 1995). Other scholars suggest that lack of motivation may prevent individuals from learning to use HIT, which exacerbates the limited use by individuals who may benefit the most from alternative healthcare interventions, such as those with low health literacy levels and less access to traditional healthcare systems (Sarkar et al., 2010).

Much work has been done to show that technology acceptance and individuals' perception that technology will be useful to them is significantly influenced by their self-efficacy (Agarwal et al., 2013; Lu et al., 2005; Rai et al., 2013). Self-efficacy is an individual's subjective perception of their own ability to perform a task (Bandura, 1994). For example, individuals who have more knowledge and confidence to self-manage their health exhibit more health-related behaviors, such as reading about drug interactions and eating healthy foods (Hibbard & Peters, 2003). Rai et al. (2013) used personal innovativeness toward mobile services (PIMS) as a proxy for self-efficacy and measured PIMS's impact on individuals' intention to use and assimilate mHealth as a substitute for traditional in-office doctor visits. Rai et al. (2013) found that PIMS had a significant influence on individuals' intention to use mHealth, even more so than an individual's perception of their health status. However, having a high PIMS (or self-efficacy to use HIT) coinciding with an individual's high perception of healthiness appeared to augment their intention to use mHealth (Rai et al., 2013). Telemedicine communications must effectively inform individuals how to perform a virtual physician visit and ease concerns that they will not have the ability to do so.

Affect is also influenced by the level of engagement a user has with HIT, which stems from the overall user experience (UX) (Chen et al., 2019; Milward et al.,

2017). The HCI community describes engagement as a state arising out of an individual's interaction with and use of a system—a quality of the user experience described in terms of difficulties; positive affect; endurability; aesthetic and sensory appeal; attention; feedback; variety/novelty; interactivity; and perceived user control (Chen et al., 2019; O'Brien & Toms, 2008). Users who have a positive emotional response during their interaction with HIT are more likely to continue to engage with the technology. Several studies demonstrate that patients' perceptions of the quality of a telemedicine service are shaped by the personal contact with the physician and other psychological factors (Demiris et al., 2003). Milward et al. (2017) report that users are more motivated to use HIT when they experience a positive experience of usability, which where those that were personally relevant and tailored to their needs. Similarly, Demiris et al. (2003) discovered that attending to patients' psychosocial needs and emotional status by demonstrating empathy and engaging with patients yielded higher levels of patient satisfaction despite experiencing technical problems during the virtual physician visit.

Trust

Trust, and its effect on users' decisions to access and use a website for information, is key to understanding how to effectively design health websites that are to be used to educate consumers and provide accurate health information (Dutta-Bergman, 2003). Trust is often conceptualized as being a users' perception that the information they access is provided by an expert, from a credible source, and is quality information (Sun et al., 2019). Trusted online sources of health information differ in terms of user demographics, health beliefs, and health-information orientation. Most individuals still express a high level of trust for information provided by to them directly from physicians rather than other sources (Dutta-Bergman, 2003, Hesse et al., 2005). Yet online health information is increasingly searched for and accessed by individuals (Cline & Haynes, 2001; Fox & Rainie, 2000). Users trust health information published, sponsored, or authored by major health institutions or physicians (Cline et al., 2001; Dutta-Bergman, 2003). However, Dutta-Bergman (2003) and Freeman et al. (2004) stress that what users deem credible depends upon the integration of several factors, such as demographics, health beliefs, tailoring of content, and initial transactions with a website (Alrubaiee, 2011; Dutta-Bergman, 2003; Freeman et al., 2004; McKnight et al., 2002). Damman et al. (2009) suggest that with the increased focus on healthcare transparency, a drift in public healthcare has been towards the goal of improving consumer health literacy and enabling individuals to make knowledgeable healthcare decisions, which is anticipated to improve individuals' overall health.

Beyond an individual's knowledge level of a health topic, desire or need to access comprehensive and detailed health information, and cognitive abilities, such as information processing abilities, mental capacity, and perception, trust in an health authority, and other individual characteristics that have usability implications include demographics and personal experiences. Hsu et al. (2014) describe these usability determinants as "self-regulating," such that there is a bidirectional and interdependent association between and among behaviors, environments, and personal experiences that affect one's health literacy, successful performance of health behaviors, and ultimately health outcomes (Dewalt et al., 2004). Individual usability determinants are intertwined by one's context of use and shaped by external factors. The next section discusses some of the key contextual factors that need to be understood in the design and delivery of HIT.

Contextual/External Determinants of Usability of HIT

To reiterate, the subjective and contextual aspects of a user interaction with HIT are often confounding variables that affect usability. Environmental factors or those associated with the context of use of a HIT, such as the time one has to perform a task, the urgency of a health situation, and social and cultural practices, have implications for usability.

Time

Time is determinant of usability (Slovic, 1982). Often individuals may access and need to use health information or telemedicine in an urgent or stressful health situation; thus, they may operate in different modes of information processing (Damman et al., 2009). When searching for health information online, with limited time, users want to see the health information clearly, at first sight, and may reject a health information website immediately if there is too much information on one page (Damman et al., 2009). Users may retreat from a website because they have difficulty understanding and interpreting complex health information or may feel overwhelmed by the amount of information on one page (Damman et al., 2009). Consumers generally only scan complex health information quickly to search for the specific information they are looking for or based on their expectations for use (Carroll et al., 1986; Eysenbach, 2005; Sillence et al., 2006). Therefore, personal relevance and trust play a key role in usability (Damman et al., 2009; Sillence et al., 2006). Such factors are central to a related and important concept: trust.

Usefulness

Regardless of which information processing mode a user employs when searching for health information online, a user's perception of whether the health information will be useful to them determines whether it gains their attention and prompts them to access the information (Davis; 1989). Sun et al. (2019) argue that perception of fitness for use is key to getting users to engage with health information. Often, users will employ both information processing modes in tandem, and may switch back and forth between the information processing routes, depending on their activity, the information they find, and their motivation (Freeman et al., 2004). For instance, users may use peripheral cues initially, and if they find information immediately, then they may use their central route to process the information, but if they perceive that the information does not meet their needs, they may return to their search results and the peripheral route of information processing (Birru et al., 2004; Freeman et al., 2004). Furthermore, it has been observed by several researchers that users do not do what they say they do (Damman et al., 2009; Eysenbach & Köhler, 2002; Silberg et al., 1997). For example, when asked, consumers impart that they assess the authority of a health information website or only access information on trusted websites, but in reality, consumers often do not even visit the home page of a health information website, and nor can they recall which website they used when accessing health information (Eysenbach et al., 2002). Overwhelmingly, there is a disparity in what consumers say they do and what they find important, and what they actually do when making a decision.

The complexity or comprehensiveness of health information is also a significant determinant of usability. Too much information can be deleterious to a user's ability to process it, creating cognitive overload (Damman et al., 2009; Hibbard et al., 1997; Slovic, 1982). For instance, users may have difficulty managing too much health information; however, providing too little information diminishes the quality of the health information and, correspondingly, the usability of the health information (Damman et al., 2009). Damman et al. (2009) observe that some users want more detailed information than health information websites provide, but recognize that negotiating the balance of providing too much information with providing too little is challenging. Impicciatore et al. (1997) found the quality of health information relating to the home management of children with fever was poor, and some websites even provided inaccurate and potentially

harmful treatment information. Often, websites recommended rectal temperature measurement, yet provided no detailed instructions for taking the temperature via this method (Impicciatore et al., 1997). Complications can occur
if parents do not perform a rectal temperature reading correctly (Impicciatore
et al., 1997). Moreover, paracetamol was the most widely recommended anti-
pyretic drug; however, few websites that recommended this treatment gave specific instructions about the dose and frequency of administration (Impicciatore
et al., 1997). Milward et al. (2017) suggest that there is a fine line between providing users with as much content as possible and tailoring content for target
users' needs when it concerns usability.

Social Dimension: Participants and Stakeholders

Healthcare does not occur in isolation, there are many stakeholders involved
in the delivery of healthcare. Patients engage in health information in a variety of contexts that include various stakeholders, such as healthcare providers,
caregivers, friends, and family (Dang et al., 2008; Goldberg et al., 2011). For
instance, Dang et al. (2008) discovered that a telephone-linked care program
designed to provide communication, support, and education to caregivers of
patients with dementia did not result in lowering the incidence of depression
among the caregivers enrolled in the program; however, the caregivers were satisfied with the support offered by the assisted technology and found it easy to
use. In Marco-Ruiz et al.'s (2017) think-aloud usability study of consumer-
oriented clinical decision support systems (CDSSs), it was discovered that users
desired options that specifically allowed them to enter information on behalf
of another person, which indicates that often health situations involve other
people. Other studies suggest that the lack of interpersonal or social aspects of
telemedicine systems, in particular those that provide remote home monitoring
or virtual physician consultations, is a major barrier to user acceptance and
adoption of telemedicine (Agnisarman et al., 2017; Alaiad & Zhou, 2017).
Jetha et al. (2011) surmise that many health information websites only provide general health information and do not consider the many stakeholders
who are involved in an individual's health situation, such as community-based
organizations and caregivers, and that these specific audiences require more specific health messages. Sarkar et al. (2010) agree that inadequate socially and culturally relevant health communications influence the use of internet-based HISs.
For instance, most physical activity information websites aimed at patients with
spinal cord injuries do not include social and cognitive approaches to motivating patients to be physically active, nor do they tailor the health information

to patients at different stages in their recovery from spinal cord injury (Jetha et al., 2011).

HIT that includes a social feature has been perceived as useful and liked by users as it allows for users to connect with others and share similar health situations, which elevates user motivation to use the HIT (Milward et al., 2017). To increase the acceptance and uptake of telemedicine, healthcare professionals and providers must be sensitive to the social and cultural aspects of healthcare and individual health contexts, and design HIT and health information that address the social and assisted living needs of patients and other stakeholders (Greenhalgh et al., 2012).

An individual's social network and relationships will sway their decision to accept and use new technology. Lu et al. (2005) found that social influences shape perceived usefulness and ease of use of wireless internet services via mobile technology (WIMT), which impact one's adoption of technology. However, internal beliefs seem to have a more powerful effect on one's intention to use new technology (Lu et al., 2005). Because both internal beliefs and social influences directly and indirectly impact technology acceptance and adoption, a variety of marketing strategies and communications should be considered to attract different users and encourage widespread diffusion of telemedicine.

Cultural Beliefs and Practices

Digital health interventions and the ability to communicate critical health information effectively on a global scale have enormous potential to improve healthcare delivery, mitigate the transmission of illnesses, and improve health outcomes overall. The rise in the delivery of eHealth, telemedicine, and other HIT to international audiences with diverse cultures requires HIT designers to determine how the context in which information is presented affects what constitutes credible information and aligns with the cultural perspectives of health and disease and medical practices. Culture plays a major role in shaping human behavior and individuals' perspectives (Khaled et al., 2006). The success of a health communication or digital health intervention depends on the degree to which it is culturally appropriate (Orji & Mandryk, 2014). St.Amant (2021) describes the three key visuals that are often used to communicate health information as the individuals who administer the care (caregivers, doctors), the objects used to administer the care (medical instruments), and the setting in which the care is administered (clinic). Designing usable HIT requires one to know what is culturally appropriate, practiced, and accepted for the target user population. For instance, Wilson et al. (2003) evaluated the usability of anticoagulation patient education materials delivered to African Americans patients in the hospital and discovered that none of the materials contained any information that recognized the healing systems, practices, and food preferences or diet restrictions unique to African Americans. For instance, anticoagulation patient education materials delivered to an African American population should specifically address the dietary patterns and desires of African Americans with respect to vitamin K foods, and should promote patients taking an active role in their disease treatment. Orji et al. (2014) analyzed North America and African cultures to be able to suggest design guidelines for digital health interventions that would be effective in changing users' behaviors and attitudes. North America was perceived as an individualistic culture and Africa was perceived as a collectivistic culture, for which Orji et al., 2014, suggested using different design. In a collectivist culture, individuals maintain tight relationships and perform behaviors in the interest of the community as a whole, whereas in an individualist culture, individuals have a self-interest and consider the individual as the determinant of their purpose and goals (Khaled et al., 2006). Including more personalized design elements for the American population would be culturally sensitive, yet including more social support features for the African population would be more effective in creating behavior change. To design a usable HIT, one must understand the culture in which one is delivering the HIT.

FORMATIVE AND SUMMATIVE USABILITY TESTING

UCD consists of several steps that are undertaken prior to implementation or delivering a final product to the intended user population. In Chapter 2, UCD was described as a four-stage process; however, these four stages are not linear and the activities that take place within each of the stages are largely dependent upon the time and resources one has to complete a technical project or develop a HIT. Moreover, UCD is considered an iterative design process, whereby the assessments and usability evaluations performed in various stages provide insight that is then used to make adjustments in the design through further iterations in order to improve usability. Once a product is finalized and delivered to the target user population or implemented in the healthcare setting in which it will be used, more and continuous testing must be done to ensure the HIT is usable and utilized.

The collection of usability assessments and testing conducted during the "design and refine" stages of UCD are termed "formative" usability testing.

Formative usability evaluations are those that are focused on identifying usability problems before a product is completed so they can be fixed prior to finalizing the product (Redish et al., 2002). Usability assessments that take place after a product has already been implemented or delivered as a final product to the intended user population and is being used in real-time are called "summative" usability testing. Often, these types of usability evaluations are termed "validation" testing because they are used to simply validate that there is a degree of usability or certify that they are being used; however, these are generally reliant on metrics that only show utility, but do not provide insight into usability. These metrics generally answer the question "Is it being used?" instead of the question "How is it being used?"

The terms "formative" and "summative" were first used by Michael Scriven (1967) when referring to the instruments and roles of curriculum evaluation. "Formative evaluations were performed during the development of the curriculum, whereas summative evaluations were conducted as a final evaluation of the project or person" (Scriven, 1967, p. 42). The HCI discipline and related fields have since adopted these terms to distinguish where in the full system design lifecycle the usability testing is taking place and how the data are used.

Formative Usability Testing Methods

There are generally more formative usability testing methods than there are summative usability testing methods, and this is revealing of the importance of usability testing to achieve the goal of usability. The summative usability testing methods discussed in this book include heuristic evaluation, cognitive walkthrough, think-aloud, and eye-tracking.

Summative Usability Testing Methods

Summative usability testing that is conducted after a final product has been released and is being used by the intended target user population is often used to confirm that a technology is being used. The raw data collected from summative usability tests are usually in the form of quantitative data. Results from summative usability testing are used to corroborate utility, and they do not identify specific usability problems, nor are they used to further refine or enhance a technology. At best, summative usability testing results are used to provide recommendations for future releases of a technology. That said, there is a place for summative usability testing to fit within a mixed-methods study, as summative usability testing can be leveraged in a long-term UCD of a HIT or used to triangulate data sets in mixed-methods studies. Summative usability testing methods are often in the form of questionnaires; those discussed in this book include the System Usability Scale (SUS), the Post-Study System Usability (PSSUQ), and the Telehealth Usability Questionnaire (TUQ).

SUMMARY

The individual and contextual factors that influence the usability of health information are important considerations when designing and delivering health information and HIT to be able to meet users' health information needs and support their changing health contexts. A multi-level framework is required to holistically analyze an audience and be able to design for usability.

To reiterate, the subjective and contextual aspects of a user interaction with HIT are often confounding variables that affect usability, but this is why mixed-methods are so valuable to be able to study multidimensions of usability and from multiple perspectives. Lastly, formative and summative usability evaluations were defined in terms of purpose and the stage of the full system development life cycle in which they typically are conducted. The next chapter will describe the mixed-methods approach and common usability inspection methods.

4

Quantitative and Qualitative Methods

INTRODUCTION

This chapter discusses quantitative and qualitative methods. First, a broad definition of each type of method will be provided, followed by identification of what types of data are obtained from using each method. Various data analysis techniques will be discussed, as will what inferences and conclusions can be made based on the findings from each method. This chapter will provide an overview of different quantitative and qualitative methods, which offers scaffolding knowledge for the next chapter on mixed-methods.

A TALE OF TWO METHODS

Quantitative and qualitative methods both make important contributions to furthering knowledge in the field of health informatics/HIT, but they differ vastly regarding the study design and insights offered. Usability studies are considered empirical research, which relies on experiential or observational data in order to extract or obtain knowledge (Mishra & Alok, 2017). Usability studies of HIT are recognized as critical to the success of the HIT implementation and intervention, yet the wide range of quantitative and qualitative usability testing methods applied to HIT make it difficult to decide on a usability assessment plan and how to measure usability. This book encourages and advocates for the use of mixed-methods, which involves the complementary use of both quantitative and qualitative methods. Before discussing mixed-methods study designs in greater detail in Chapter 5, the distinctions between quantitative and qualitative methods will be clarified in this chapter.

DOI: 10.1201/9781003460886-4

It is common for industry professionals and those without an academic background to use the terms "methodology" and "method" interchangeably. However, they do not have the same meaning. The types of methods one uses in their study are dependent on their methodology, which is based on one's ontological and epistemological perspective. For scholars and those in academia, when investigating a problem or developing research questions, ontology and epistemology are important considerations that determine how one approaches their research inquiry, including their methodology and the methods they use to collect data. It is likely that UX research professionals who have received their education and training from UX bootcamps or online courses have only been introduced to methods, which are the ways in which data is collected and analyzed, including data collection instruments, tools, and techniques. UX professionals from this background have never had to consider where their beliefs, values, and assumptions about reality and knowledge lie within different research paradigms (Guba & Lincoln, 1996; Kuhn, 1962). There are various research paradigms (e.g., positivism, interpretivism, constructivism) (Howell, 2013) that offer frameworks for human inquiry, but they will not be discussed in this book. The basic philosophical terminology will be introduced here.

Ontology is the study of the nature of being or reality (what it means to exist) (Howell, 2013). Epistemology deals with the nature of knowledge; it is the study of what is considered knowledge and how one goes about discovering knowledge (Howell, 2013). Ontology and epistemology are tied together, and these philosophical positions underpin methodologies, "which in turn identify rationales for specific methods of data collection" (Howell, 2013, Preface). Methodology is defined as the research strategy that outlines how one goes about undertaking a research project; it involves an understanding of the methods used in your field and the theories or principles behind them in order to develop an approach that matches your research objectives (Howell, 2013). Methods, on the other hand, are the specific tools and procedures used to collect and analyze data—for example, experiments, surveys, interviews, observations, and statistical tests. Mixed-methods is a methodology that adheres to the concept of methodological pluralism, which is the understanding that using multiple and different methods to collect a variety of data sets allows one to better study and understand complex problems. In more modern terms, scholars and UX researchers fall in the middle of the various ontological and epistemological viewpoints; therefore, mixed-methods has become a valuable methodology in the social sciences, including technical communication, UX, and HCI.

Quantitative Methods

In the humanities, as well as the natural and social sciences, quantitative methods emerged from the positivist paradigm, which assumes that true knowledge can only be discovered, or phenomena can only be explained, by performing experiments with tightly controlled variables resulting in measurable outcomes (Ahmad et al., 2019). Under these assumptions, the nature of scientific inquiry was objective and systematic, and thus held a high degree of rigor and replicability because it was based on the aspect of quantity or extent, which can be measured accurately and precisely (Ahmad et al., 2019; Mishra et al., 2017).

In short, quantitative methods comprise any type of study or experiment that yields numerical results or statistical data, which can be used to draw conclusions. Quantitative methods are valuable when one wants to generalize results to larger populations or use statistical data, such as frequencies or percentages, to support predictions. Validation testing, benchmarking, and competitive comparisons are goals for performing quantitative usability testing. Quantitative usability testing is often performed in the summative stages of UCD because findings are used as evidence that a HIT is or is not usable, or provide an overall rating of usability that can be generalized to the target users.

Quantitative Usability Research Inquires: Methods & Data Analysis

Because the type of data that is collected when using quantitative methods is based in numerical metrics or values, the research questions they help to answer drive the study design decisions and help determine how best to collect and analyze the data. Quantitative methods are valuable when one wants to demonstrate that a HIT is or is not usable by the representative population based on some sort of quantifiable usable metric, like task completion success, frequency of errors, or overall usability questionnaires that result in user satisfaction scores. Usability evaluations that focus on efficiency or effectiveness are often conducted using quantitative methods. Any usability study that measures usability using a predefined metric, numerical value, or figure would be considered a quantitative usability study. Quantitative research answers the questions of how many or how much because they are objective measurements that can be captured. Quantitative findings are also used to make estimations or predictions about future frequency, magnitude, or incidence of the phenomenon under investigation (Curry et al., 2009). There are various types of quantitative data that can be collected to evaluate or determine whether a product has a sufficient level of usability. Below is a list of some of the more common usability metrics that could be measured using quantitative methods:

- Task completion success rates—Percentage of subjects who completed tasks successfully (Campbell et al., 2021; Georgsson & Staggers, 2016)
- Task completion times—Average amount of time for subjects to complete tasks.
- Error rates—Number of errors subjects encountered during their interaction.
- User satisfaction—Typically, user satisfaction is a subjective perception that cannot be quantified; however, a Brooke (1986) developed a quantified metric of user satisfaction that can be measuring using the System Usability Scale (SUS). The SUS provides a single score that has been reliably used to demonstrate the overall usability of a system.
- Questionnaires or surveys that result in ratings—Likert scales are often used to psychometrically measure users' impression of system usability.
- Eye-tracking metrics—Fixations and saccades are gaze points and patterns that are measured during eye-tracking tests.
- Number of mouse clicks—This figure represents the degree of efficiency a user interface (UI) allows for users to navigate to specific information.
- Cost efficiency—Monetary expenditures required for

Because quantitative findings are used primarily to verify that a HIT has sufficient usability or the usability of previous versions has been refined and improved, usability attributes are determined on the basis of the user profile, context of use, and other subjective and contextual factors that may affect usability, then a performance level is set for each attribute (Jokela et al., 2006). Benchmarking is the process of evaluating each version of a design and comparing it with previous versions. A quantifiable usability metric is defined and usability testing is conducted on prototypes or early versions of a technology, and again after iterative changes have been made or on refined versions of the technology. Any improvement in that metric following validation testing is considered an improvement in usability. For instance, if 80 percent of users were able to successfully complete tasks in the first round of usability testing, and 90 percent of users were able to successfully complete tasks in the second round of usability testing, this would be considered an improvement in usability. A quantified usability target is sometimes defined in the early stages of the full system design lifecycle and later tested against this requirement in the later stages of the full system design lifecycle. Validation testing is conducted after a HIT has already been implemented in the clinical setting or context for which it was intended and in which is being used. Validation testing is done to provide evidence that a HIT has sufficient usability.

Sample Sizes

Quantitative research aims for large sample populations, which is considered to increase the reliability of the study. Maramba et al.'s (2019) scoping review of usability studies of eHealth discovered that sample size is not given much attention or reported on in most usability tests of eHealth applications. Yet sample size is an important consideration when designing a quality study. Specifically when employing quantitative methods, sample size is a study design decision that must be reported clearly and justified. Larger sample sizes allow researchers to better determine the average values of their data and avoid skewed results that can occur when testing a small number of possibly atypical samples (Ahmad et al., 2019).

Large sample sizes between 100 and 450 subjects have been used to collect quantitative usability data using questionnaires (Maramba et al, 2019). Sample size selections in usability investigations are also determined by the resources available and by the feasibility. Data analysis is usually performed using mathematical computations or generating statistics such as percentages or sums and reported as such.

Quantitative usability research is needed to be able to illustrate return on investment (ROI) or to demonstrate that a previous design has been improved; however, it does not pinpoint specific usability problems or distinguish what or where in a UI creates problems for users during their interaction. Thus, qualitative research is the primary usability testing approach adopted in health informatics, given the human factors involved in the usability of HIT and the ability of qualitative research to specifically identify social, cognitive, physical, cultural, and context-of-use factors that impact usability (Borycki, 2011; Borycki & Kushniruk, 2010; Kushniruk et al., 2005; Morgan 1998; Redish & Lowry, 2010).

Qualitative Methods

Qualitative methods are used to deeply evaluate complex phenomena and seek to gain an in-depth understanding of the human experience of the particular phenomena under investigation. As such, the data gained from qualitative methods are largely unstructured and the insight gained are based on researchers' inferences and interpretations of the data. Qualitative methods involved the direct assessment of a user interacting with technology or the HIT under evaluation or the collection of subjective data from human subjects acting as representative users of the HIT under investigation. Qualitative methods include any type of method that collects data that is unquantifiable, such as complexity, breadth, or range of occurrences or phenomena (Curry et al., 2009). Every individual and health situation is different and unique because individuals have various personal characteristics and contextual aspects that affect usability. This makes understanding how representative users of a target population interact with HIT a critical part of user-centered design and the patient-centered design focus in HIT. Just as UCD seeks to optimize the user's ability to achieve goals by interacting with technology, which enhances UX, patient-centered HIT seeks to optimize the patient-experience of healthcare from access, delivery, treatment, and knowledge of health information through technology that is usable (Al Muammar et al., 2018; Wilson, 2009). Qualitative research seeks to understand how users interact with HIT and identify the root cause of usability problems. Findings from quantitative data analysis are used to improve the usability of HIT.

Qualitative Usability Research Inquiries: Methods and Data Analysis

Qualitative methods include any study, test, or protocol that collects unstructured data in the form of notes, reports, video, and audio data generated from observations and the verbal or written reports from subjects. Various types of qualitative methods are used in usability studies, and the data collection techniques and analyses are not linked to any one paradigm or framework because they are determined by the research inquiry and the resources available for the research to take place. The following are some of the common qualitative methods applied in usability studies of HIT:

- *Ethnographic research.* Observational method that collects field notes and quotes from representative users in order to understand their needs and interactions with HIT.
- *Interviews/focus groups.* User research that collects verbal reports from representative users of their experiences with HIT.
- *Cognitive walkthroughs.* Subject matter experts (SMEs) simulate target users' interactions with HIT to discover usability problems.

- *Heuristic evaluations.* SMEs evaluate HIT against a set of usability heuristics, such as Nielsen's (1994) 10 usability heuristics (visibility of system status, match between system and the real world, user control and freedom, etc.).
- *Think-alouds.* Representative users perform representative tasks using HIT and speak their thoughts aloud in an attempt to describe why they are doing what they are doing.

Qualitative data have to be interpreted by the researcher. Data analysis of qualitative data is conducted in ways that make sense for the researcher and help them answer their research questions. Qualitative data are often inductively coded into themes that emerge from the data or deductively coded according to a previously established framework (Hsieh & Shannon, 2005). Findings from qualitative data are often inferences made by the researcher as they are able to make them using a theoretical lens or through application.

Because qualitative findings are used primarily to be able to improve the usability of HIT during the iterative design process, large sample sizes are not required, nor are they cost-effective. Nielsen and Landauer (1993) demonstrate that only five users are required to reveal 85 percent of the usability problems in a think-aloud usability evaluation. Only four or five subjects are needed to find 80 percent of the usability problems (Virzi, 1992); therefore, the "five participant" target number has been standardized. That said, given users' range of differences, the notion that any five representative users can discover 80 percent of the major usability flaws is overrated, as Faulkner (2003) demonstrates that the average percentage of usability problems found by any one set of five users can range from 55 percent to about 95 percent. However, to reinstate Nielsen's point about the five-user rule, the number of usability problems or severity of the usability problems that are discovered as you test more users may not be cost-effective. Data saturation—or the identification of any new usability problems—may be reached by the fifth user you test (Nielsen, 2000).

Each qualitative method used has been associated to require a specific number of users (Alroobaea & Mayhew, 2014), but all sample sizes used in qualitative research are smaller than what is required in quantitative research because the goal is to identify specifics (usability problems, contextual aspects, user perception), not to generalize to a wider population.

Whereas qualitative data are "known" to be less rigorous because the data are analyzed using inferences by the researcher, they can contain biases or have a lower degree of reliability because each researcher may be subject to interpreting qualitative data differently. However, the major affordance of qualitative methods is that they are able to identify specific usability issues that can be used to make design recommendations or communicate to designers to be able to refine the design of a HIT in order to make it more usable. The ability to pinpoint usability problems in a HIT, such as a poor navigation menu or a font size that is too small, is why quantitative methods are generally performed and more valuable in the formative stages of UCD because design iterations can be done prior to the release of the HIT to the intended user population.

SUMMARY

Quantitative methods include any type of experiment that yields numerical results, whereas qualitative methods collect unstructured, observational, and subjective data, and are open to interpretation by the researcher during data analysis. While both quantitative and qualitative methods make important contributions to usability studies, qualitative methods are the primary method in mixed-methods studies because their findings are directly applied to improve the usability of HIT. Because only one quality of usability is able to be evaluated using any one method alone, regardless of whether quantitative or qualitative methods are used solely, the motivation for combining qualitative and quantitative methods in a mixed-methods study comes from the ability to collect a compilation of usability metrics and gain a more holistic, comprehensive understanding of usability. Additionally, as will be discussed in the next chapter, the affordances of any one method offset the limitations of another; likewise, the strengths of one method can enhance the performance of another, and finally, researchers can corroborate their conclusions with evidence from multiple data sets.

5

Mixed-Methods Study Design and Rigor

INTRODUCTION

This chapter defines mixed-methods studies and provides a framework for designing mixed-methods studies in health informatics. The affordances and limitations of conducting mixed-methods studies are discussed. Finally, the chapter ends by explaining how the quality of a study is evaluated. Common markers of scientific rigor will be defined, such as generalizability, validity, and fidelity, as well as different approaches to ensure rigor in quantitative and qualitative research.

MIXED-METHODS STUDY DESIGN

Mixed-methods studies involve the use of more than one research method to examine the phenomenon under investigation. Mixed-methods studies may include the application of more than one method to collect multiple sets of quantitative and qualitative data to obtain a rich data corpus. Mixed-methods usability studies employ both quantitative and qualitative methods; however, one method is generally considered the primary method, and the other the secondary method (Schoonenbloom & Johnson, 2017). Generally, during UCD, which includes usability testing, qualitative methods will be the primary method used and secondary qualitative metrics may also be captured to be able to generalize to broader audiences and corroborate findings from qualitative methods with statistical data. Formative usability evaluations usually collect qualitative data because the findings are intended to be applied to iterative design changes that improve the usability of the HIT under investigation. Summative usability evaluations, in contrast, are performed after a HIT has been released to the target

DOI: 10.1201/9781003460886-5

user and are intended to generate numbers that are supposed to confirm that the HIT is usable; therefore, they collect quantitative data. Johnson et al. (2007, p. 123) offer the following operational definition of mixed-methods studies:

> The type of research in which a researcher or team of researchers combines elements of qualitative and quantitative research approaches (e. g., use of qualitative and quantitative viewpoints, data collection, analysis, inference techniques) for the broad purposes of breadth and depth of understanding and corroboration.

The unique distinguishing factor of mixed-methods studies is that multiple methods are applied within the confines of a single study. That said, various study designs]could be used to structure a mixed-methods study. Of course, with all studies there are affordances and limitations, but the affordances of mixed-methods studies far outweigh the limitations. Additionally, despite the positivist perspective that only quantitative research can be conducted with extreme rigor because qualitative research can be compromised by researcher biases, misinterpretations, and unstructured data (Cypress, 2017), by applying multiple qualitative and quantitative methods and employing several quality assurance strategies, mixed-methods scientific research can be considered to have a high degree of scientific rigor.

Affordances of Mixed-Methods Studies

There are several affordances of mixed-methods studies relating to the ways in which usability can be evaluated, data can be interpreted, and findings can be triangulated.

Adopting a mixed-methods approach to study design enables multiple data sets to be obtained, creating a rich data corpus that can be analyzed and interpreted from different perspectives. Using more than one method to evaluate and measure the same construct allows the triangulation of data and can generate rich insights that may not be obtained through the use of only one method (Alaiad et al., 2017). Triangulation refers to the collection of data from multiple sources in order to obtain a rich data corpus and generate the ability to make comparisons across data sets (Creswell, 2002; Golafshani, 2003). Triangulation optimizes the quality and rigor of research (Creswell, 2002; Golafshani, 2003). Furthermore, by using different techniques for the same inquiry, the limitations of one method may be offset by the advantages of another (Kushniruk et al., 2001). For instance, when performing empirical research, humans may be subject to memory loss and recall deficiencies regarding the phenomena of inquiry, but by performing multiple methods, such as interviews to understand users' needs, usability testing to evaluate user performance and identify design flaws in the HIT, and retrospective questionaries to understand users' perceived usability, researchers are able to gain a more accurate perception of the subjective user experience.

Several variables are able to be observed in mixed-methods studies, as well as how each relates to the phenomenon under investigation. Lastly, prolonged engagement with data allows researchers to intimately analyze qualitative data and make meaningful interpretations.

Limitations of Mixed-Methods Studies

No study is without limitations, and there are a few drawbacks of mixed-methods studies. Because mixed-methods studies involve conducting multiple methods examining one or more constructs, they are often onerous and time-consuming. Additionally, depending on what methods and tools utilized to conduct various methods, mixed-methods studies can be costly.

Researchers may require the expertise of other disciplines, which is why collaboration is encouraged, but tools that afford collaborative data analysis and the ability to store, manage, and organize a vast amount of data, such as data analysis software, like QSR International's NVivo 12 qualitative data analysis software (QSR International n.d.), can be costly (Maher et al., 2018).

Furthermore, because multiple methods are being applied in a mixed-methods study, either sequentially or simultaneous, mixed-methods studies are complex, complicated, onerous, and resource-intensive. An interdisciplinary team may collaborate to contribute the subject matter expertise of each member, and automation and data analysis tools may be leveraged to support the integration of data and collaborative data analysis, as well as hasten processes, yet these processes too can be expensive.

Methodological Diversity

Methodological pluralism is argued to fuel creative investigations, whereby methods used can complement one another to craft a cumulative body of knowledge (Alaiad et al., 2017; Slife & Gantt, 1999; Venkatesh et al., 2013). Mixed-methods study designs afford methodological diversity (Venkatesh et al., 2013), and for this reason embrace interdisciplinary collaborations. Kushniruk et al. (2004) argue that as the field of health informatics becomes more complex and more essential for patient-centered healthcare (Schmidt-Kraepelin et al., 2014), it is necessary to evolve usability studies of HIT to address HIT usability problems that impact patient safety (Alotaibi & Federico, 2017; Kushniruk et al., 2010) and health disparities (Gibbons et al., 2014; Goldberg et al., 2011), and improve the healthcare experience (Campbell, 2020c) with evidence-based approaches.

RIGOR: EVALUATING THE QUALITY OF QUANTITATIVE AND QUALITATIVE RESEARCH

What is meant by scientific rigor? The term "rigor" emerged from the positivist tradition that maintains that scientific research is conducted in order to produce universal laws and knowledge that govern observable phenomena (Delmar, 2010; Golafshani, 2003; Marquart, 2017). As such, scientific rigor refers to the soundness, exactitude, and accuracy of a study's design and methodological approach, including planning, constructs tested, measurements, data collection instruments, analysis, and reporting (Marquart, 2017).

Quantitative and qualitative forms of research are fundamentally different in their ability to establish rigor. This distinction between the ways in which quantitative research and qualitative research establish scientific rigor stems from the fact that quantitative methods are rooted in the positive perspective, which reports investigative findings as numerical information that objectively establish truth about scientific phenomena. Qualitative results have no standardized reporting mechanism and are often derived from the subjective interpretations of unstructured data or inferences made by the researcher. Qualitative research stems from a social constructivist paradigm, which maintains that humans construct knowledge based on their interactions with other humans and their environment, and thus naturalistic inquiry seeks to understand phenomena in context-specific settings in which the researcher does not attempt to manipulate the phenomenon of interest: "It is difficult to express rigor when human attributes and variables are so dynamic and change depending on the context" (Cypress, 2017, p. 256). Moreover, given that usability studies in health informatics focus on understanding the human factors involved in the interaction with HIT, the dynamics and various cognitive-socio-technical-cultural aspects that affect usability are unique and difficult to measure, depending on the target user and context of use. Thus, empirical research using qualitative methods is better suited to investigating real user activities, which are unique for each individual and inherently impacted by contextual factors. Knowledge from qualitative research is not constructed from standardized formulas, but from the inferences made by researchers or from real end-users who participate in usability testing. As such, qualitative research is assumed to be imbued with biases and is unreliable. This often polemic debate between the level of rigor that can be established by quantitative and qualitative methods is largely due to the difference in quality indicators and how they are evaluated. Although both quantitative and qualitative methods utilize similar criteria to establish rigor, they differ in their approach to determine and demonstrate quality indicators, such as generalizability, reliability, and validity.

Because quantitative research is based on numbers, which are calculated using systematic, objective methods, quantitative research has traditionally been recognized as being more scientifically rigorous than qualitative research, and common quality indicators (reliability and validity) have been operationalized. Critics of qualitative research argue that research is based on mere subjective anecdotal evidence riddled with bias, and that it lacks reproducibility (Mays & Pope, 1995). Furthermore, given that qualitative research designs are often flexible and emergent in nature, there is no standard or universal approach to demonstrating rigor (Cypress, 2017). That said, qualitative research plays an important and essential role in the health and medical field, technical communication, and most certainly in investigations of usability of HIT because findings are valued for their ability to be applied in the refinement and redesign of HIT to improve usability. As such, qualitative research can be considered to have a higher degree of pragmatism because qualitative methods are performed in order to be able to obtain useful, practical insight. Furthermore, HCI and HIT usability practitioners and designers do not hold qualitative research studies to the same standards of rigor as those who subscribe to purely quantitative research because usability studies examine the human, the HIT user interface, and their interaction, and most often collect qualitative data to be analyzed, made sense of, and transformed into useful information. In the health sciences, qualitative research is arguably more imperative because the consequences are greater when human lives are affected, and the findings are more valuable if used to improve the design of HIT that is going to be efficacious.

It is therefore important to define how different methodological approaches are evaluated in terms of rigor and to prime researchers with an understanding of the terminology that will be used to discuss the soundness and integrity of a mixed-methods study because they involve both quantitative and qualitative methods. Table 5.1 summarizes quality indicators and attributes of rigor commonly used to evaluate research and how each type of research method defines and approaches demonstrating scientific rigor.

Table 5.1 illustrates that often different, but similar, attributes of quality are used to express scientific rigor in qualitative studies than in quantitative studies. Given that mixed-methods studies combine qualitative and quantitative methods, the field of health and medicine has established best practices rather

TABLE 5.1

Scientific rigor indicators, definition, and demonstration techniques used in quantitative and qualitative research

Quality indicator	Quantitative research definition	Qualitative research definition
Reliability	[*Reproducibility*] Refers to the extent to which the methods (and data collection instruments) used in a study can be replicated and achieve the same, consistent results. Statistical significance may be used to establish reliability in a quantitative study. Inferential statistics look at the measured statistics, the sample size, and the variability of the data and calculate the probability of that statistic being unusual. Confidence levels are used to determine the degree to which one's findings are predictive of real-life scenarios—meaning what level of probability would make the researcher confident that if they repeated the study, it would generate the same results. Common confidence level values are 90 per cent and 95 percent. Interrater reliability is another common metric used to establish that a study's methods are reliable. Interrater reliability refers to the extent to which two or more researchers' inferences agree with one another. Chapter 6 discusses interrater reliability in more detail; however, several metrics are used to express interrater reliability: percentage agreement; Cohen's kappa (when there are only two raters); the Fleiss kappa (when there are three or more raters); the contingency coefficient; the Pearson r and the Spearman Rho; the intra-class correlation coefficient; the concordance correlation coefficient; and Krippendorff's alpha. Each metric has its own scale that expresses low to high interrater reliability.	*Accuracy, authority of research,* and *dependability* are often replacement terms used in qualitative research. Qualitative research establishes reliability by clearly describing the systematic methods used, defining and operationalizing variables and measurements, and demonstrating reflexivity. Reflexivity refers to assessment of the influence of the investigator's own background, perceptions, and interests on the qualitative research process. Acknowledging one's own biases, providing rich descriptions, clearly and accurately representing participants' perspectives, and obtaining peer reviews are hallmarks to establishing reliability.

TABLE 5.1 (Continued)

Scientific rigor indicators, definition, and demonstration techniques used in quantitative and qualitative research

Quality indicator	Quantitative research definition	Qualitative research definition
Validity	The accuracy and precision of the findings as they relate to the phenomenon being studied. *Generalizability* is similarly defined as the degree in which the findings from one study can be applied to other contexts, groups, or settings. Quantitative research generally establishes validity by simply using large sample populations and recruiting from clearly defined populations. There are various dimensions of validity: • *Internal validity* concerns whether the attribute or variable one has chosen to measure is really an accurate measurement of the phenomenon under investigation. • *External validity* is the degree to which the measurements or observations in the test environment are applicable to the phenomenon in real life. • *Ecological validity* is the extent to which the context of the study and circumstances under which subjects are evaluated match their real-world, natural setting and the activities subjects would normally carry out. • *Predictive validity* is the extend in which the criteria measured on a test matches a test subject's actual experience or behaviors.	*Trustworthiness, credibility, applicability*, and *transferability* are interchangeable with validity and generalizability in qualitative research. Effective strategies for establishing [validity] applicability and trustworthiness include: prolonged and intimate engagement with data, use of qualitative data analysis tools, member checking, external audits, and triangulation. Another way by which qualitative researchers express that their findings are generalizable is by demonstrating that their findings are only generalizable to certain groups or contexts and/or demonstrating reference to a body of literature. This is referred to as *contextualization*.

Sources: Cronbach & Meehl, 1955; Cropley, 2019; Cypress, 2017; Golafshani, 2003; Hughes, 1999; Krefting, 1991; Kushniruk et al., 2013; Lincoln & Guba, 1985; Long & Johnson, 2000; Maher et al., 2018; Mays et al., 1995; McHugh, 2012; Meyrick, 2006; Nielsen, 1993a; Noble & Smith, 2015; Ruby, 1980; Winter, 2000.

than using strict criteria to demonstrate that a mixed-methods study has been conducted with a sufficient, if not high, level of scientific rigor. For instance, rather than using a calculated confidence level to determine that a quantitative study's results are highly likely to be accurate, the results of a qualitative study can exhibit trustworthiness by clearly describing the study design and rationale for leveraging such methods, clearly listing the steps taken to collect and analyze data, displaying ethics in research design and attempts to avoid or minimize error or bias (Cypress, 2017; Johnson et al., 2020).

Triangulation

Optimization of research methods is achieved through triangulation. Triangulation refers to the collection of data from multiple sources in order to obtain a rich data corpus and have the ability to make comparisons across data sets; this ultimately improves the rigor (Creswell, 2002; Golafshani, 2003; Mays et al., 1995). Triangulation can occur by engaging with multimodal data, including various data sets that can be obtained from quantitative and qualitative data collection instruments, such as textual, video, and statistical data. Maher et al. (2018) achieved a high level of rigor by collecting various data sets from interviews, affinity diagraming, and observations. Maher et al. (2018, p. 12) argue that triangulation enables researchers to:

> "immerse" themselves in data, to explore all the possible nuances and relationships, to view data from a variety of perspectives, and to move from micro- to macroview, in order to This form of analysis is augmented by multimodality forms of interaction with the data.

Triangulation can also be achieved when researchers compare two or more data sets, as Khajouei et al. (2017) did when comparing the frequencies and categories of identified usability problems discovered when using two different methods: heuristic evaluation or cognitive walkthrough. Numerous scholars contend that mixed-methods research is a successful way to triangulate data (Bryant et al., 2008; Fonteyn et al., 1993; Peute et al., 2015a; Wolpin et al., 2015) and can strengthen and enrich results.

Fidelity and Pragmaticism

Other attributes that are associated with quality usability studies in health informatics include *fidelity* and *pragmaticism*. These are both important considerations when designing usability studies because they view the study or experiment setting and the ability of the research to be executed on the basis of resources available and other constraints.

Fidelity refers to the degree in which the research setting mimics or simulates the context in which a user would interact with technology and how the user would interact with the technology (Kushniruk, 2002; Kushniruk et al., 2013). Fidelity is one of the most important considerations in the design and execution of empirical research and involves two dimensions: the testing setting/environment and the HCI interactions with the technology or system under investigation.

The testing environment and representative HCI interactions can range from low-fidelity to high-fidelity simulations (See Figure 5.1).

In UCD, low-fidelity prototypes or study settings may be used to obtain baseline information about the user interaction in the beginning stages of the full system design lifecycle—to understand the target users and technology specifications. High-fidelity usability testing may be conducted in the end stages of UCD to identify design flaws that can iteratively be refined to optimize usability before the final release of the technology. Depending on the stage in which one is performing usability testing, high-fidelity environments may be more suitable because the more the user interaction with HIT resembles a real-life scenario, the more the findings will be able to be used to make accurate predictions about how the intended user population will use the HIT to achieve specified goals in real life.

Dowding et al. (2019) created low-fidelity paper prototypes of EHR dashboards intended to be used by home healthcare nurses to have nurse participants provide rapid feedback that they then used to make iterative design changes to an EHR dashboard in development. The low-fidelity prototypes offered a low-cost model of the dashboard with which participants could interact to provide value and useful feedback in the beginning of the full system design lifecycle.

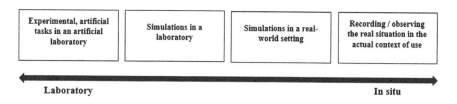

FIGURE 5.1
Spectrum of low-fidelity testing environments to high-fidelity testing environments. The greater the fidelity, the greater the likelihood that the testing environment and user interaction resemble a real-life context of use.

High-fidelity usability testing settings include naturalistic environments, like in situ—in the real-world environment in which users would interact with the HIT under investigation. Kushniruk (2002) insists that when attempting to generalize how usable a HIT is to complex real-world situations, such as when an individual experiences poor health, controlling for all factors that may occur in real-world situations is not desirable. In-situ testing environments are favorable at the end of the full system design lifecycle because they offer a more realistic and accurate representation of how the target end user actually interacts with HIT to be achieve their goals for use. A high-fidelity usability study of a medication administration system was carried out at a hospital and interfaced with technologies it would be required to use when implemented in the hospital (Borycki et al., 2011).

Fidelity may also refer to the simulated interactions a subject might perform with a HIT in a usability study. Vignettes are often used to describe situations or scenarios that subjects are asked to imagine, in which they perform interactions with HIT as if they were in that real-life situation. For instance, Luger et al. (2014) developed two illness vignettes that depicted the symptoms of an acute health condition that were read to participants prior to asking participates interact with an online diagnosis platform in order to understand how older adults interacted with online diagnosis platforms to correctly self-diagnose. Similarly, I developed three illness vignettes describing the types of symptoms patients would likely experience when ill and seeking telemedicine from one of three different telemedicine platforms to be able to identify usability errors encountered by subjects during their interactions (Campbell, 2020a).

High-fidelity simulations can be used by developing representative tasks that the users of HIT are expected to undertake when using the system and having usability testing subjects attempt to perform such tasks. For example, in a study of errors induced by use of a medication order entry system, this may include presenting representative subjects (physicians) with written descriptions of patient cases (such as a prescription list for the patient in the case) (Borycki et al., 2005). It is an imperative when selecting the representative tasks that subjects are expected to undertake that they include the tasks and activities that most emulate what users would do if in that situation in real life (Borycki et al., 2005; Kushniruk et al., 2004; Kushniruk et al., 1997; Kushniruk & Patel, 2005; Kushniruk et al., 2008; Kushniruk et al., 2010; Russ et al., 2010; Russ et al., 2018).

Pragmaticism or *utility* is the idea that the study is relevant and that it will be useful to the real world. Mann et al. (2018) argue that academically oriented usability studies value scientific rigor over studies that generate useful knowledge which can be applied in a real-world setting or situation, which result from pragmatic usability studies. A study that prioritized *pragmaticism* would leverage cost-effective, low-fidelity prototyping (Nielsen, 1989, 1994b) and quick methods to obtain real end-user feedback (Brooke, 1986) to inform rapid, agile development lifecycles, such as those used during UCD.

As healthcare systems continue to adopt more complex HIT, such as EHRs, mHealth apps, and other digital health interventions, more emphasis is put on supporting design decisions with evidence from formative usability testing (Li et al., 2012; Borycki et al., 2013) and involving end-users in the design process to contribute design recommendations and act as usability test subjects. The American Recovery and Reinvestment Act (ARRA), enacted by the U.S. Congress in February 2009, and the Health Information Technology for Economic and Clinical Health Act of 2009 (HITECH) mandate that vendors abide by the meaning use rule, perform usability testing, and engage in the certification process for EHR technology (Redish et al., 2010). The Office of the National Coordinator of Health Information Technology (ONC) certification criteria stipulates minimal usability requirements to demonstrate that HIT has sufficient usability, yet offer no standard framework for usability testing, which leads to a lack of consistent evidence-based HIT being implemented in real-life settings.

A pragmatic usability study supports these research objectives and supports the implementation of evidence-based, meaningful use HIT. Mann et al. (2018) draw attention to the disparate aims of academic and pragmatic research. Albeit using similar methods, academic research may be focused more on scientific rigor and generating large amounts of data to analyze in order to support overall conclusions. Pragmatic usability studies, however, are designed to generate quick, specific insights about usability that are used to inform product iterations that will improve usability. As a result of these conflicting priorities, academic usability studies value conducting usability studies that can demonstrate scientific rigor and are often funded by grants. Pragmatic usability studies are often performed under time constraints and have a limited budget, yet they are performed in order to gain real end-user feedback and identify usability problems that can inform agile development of successive HIT designs.

Technical communicators and usability/UX practitioners agree that UCD, which involves participation from intended users of the product, is the optimal way to design usable, customized HIT interventions that attain a high user acceptance and utilization, as well as improve public health, especially for vulnerable, underserved populations (Brunner et al., 2017; Parmar, 2010; Rose, 2016; Rose et al., 2017).

Efforts to develop effective technology tools to support evidence-based healthcare require an approach to systematic usability research that addresses both the pragmatic as well as academic needs of a project. UCD, which involves a mixed-methods framework, best contributes to the successful widespread delivery and adoption of effective HIT. The mixed-methods usability study framework I outline next achieves academic research objectives and has real-world positive health implications.

FRAMEWORK FOR DESIGNING A RIGOROUS MIXED-METHODS STUDY

In order to establish a high level of scientific rigor, yet still garner useful insights, and balance meeting academic and pragmatic research agendas, I have formulated a framework that can be used to design a high-quality mixed-methods usability study. The mixed-methods framework I outline below can be applied to any HIT usability study.

1. Develop your research questions. What insight do you want to gain by evaluating usability? How will you apply your findings? What are the implications of your study?
2. Define the usability variables of inquiry. What qualities, dimensions, or processes do you want to evaluate?
3. Identify usability metrics. How will you measure usability? What data will you collect? Will you collect quantitative or qualitative data? How will you analyze the data? How do you consider usability success?
4. Select the most suitable, feasible, and valuable usability testing methods that will allow you to capture the usability metrics you desire.
5. Use, reuse, modify, innovate usability testing methods that are best suited for your object of analysis.

Because every usability study must take into consideration the representative target users and the environment in which they are likely to interact with the product, every usability study is arguably unique and requires a unique design. Additionally, the accessibility of different resources and tools needed to execute a mixed-methods study varies by researcher, facility, and user population, so feasibility must be factored into the framework. You might want to conduct a high-fidelity usability study with a high sample population of representative users, but may not have access to a clinical setting, or you may not have the funds to reward participation, or even have access to a high number of willing participants, so you have to select methods and instruments that will allow you to achieve your study's objectives, yet be within the limits of your resources and timeframe. By identifying each component of the framework I provided, researchers, healthcare professionals, and HIT practitioners can design rigorous usability studies and achieve pragmatic objectives.

Ethics in Healthcare Research

In the health and medical field, for example, access to patients to act as subjects is limited. In addition, there are several approvals one might need to obtain prior to performing research in a clinical setting. Furthermore, often getting physicians and other stakeholders' buy-in that usability testing is essential challenges practitioners in health informatics and other professionals. These are all considerations on which a researcher must weigh in when making study design decisions, such as how to recruit subjects, how many subjects are necessary, and where the study should be conducted. Furthermore, researchers must consider the impact their study might have on participants and make ethical decisions—those that do the least harm or have the least effect on their human subjects, yet gain the most value. The ethics involved in a usability study often involve balancing priorities or research objectives with subjects' availability and needs.

The ethical considerations of performing human subjects research, which usability studies involve, must be considered both in academic and pragmatic usability investigations. Human subjects research will need to be submitted through an academic institution's Institutional Review Board (IRB) for approval and informed consent must be gained. See Appendix A for a sample informed consent form. In accordance with federal law §46.116(a)(5)(i) and (ii), five key pieces of information are required for both verbal and written informed consent. These five key pieces of information must be clear, concise, and project-specific:

1. Consent being sought for research, with participation voluntary
2. Purpose of the research, the expected duration of the prospective subject's participation, and the procedures to be followed
3. Reasonably foreseeable risks or discomforts to the prospective subject
4. Benefits to the prospective subject or to others that may reasonably be expected form the research
5. Appropriate alternative procedures or courses of treatment, if any, that might be advantageous to the prospective subject.

Written informed consent may be required for human subjects research that is approved by your IRB. Verbal informed consent only may be required for human subjects research that is classified as exempt from the requirements of the Federal Policy for the Protection of Humans Subjects because it qualifies as no risk or minimal risk to subjects. Even if you think your study qualifies for an exemption from human subjects research requirements, you still have to submit your research through your IRB for an exemption determination. Additionally, if your study is being conducted in situ or at a hospital or clinic, you will likely need to have your study approved by the specific institution, hospital, or other healthcare facility where you are conducting your research. Other ethical considerations concern the human subjects of your study. Specific populations, such as Native American and Alaska Native people, have tribal organizations that also require you to have your study approved.

Healthcare research necessitates that you do the most good while doing the least harm. Academics and practitioners who strive to understand the user experience of HIT and seek to improve the usability of HIT through user-centered research have the best intentions in mind and take into account the ethical implications of their study.

SUMMARY

This chapter defined a mixed-methods study as a study that involves the use of more than one method of examining the phenomenon under investigation, including at least one qualitative method and one quantitative method. Mixed-methods usability studies afford the ability to collect multiple data sets and analyze qualitative data in rich and meaningful ways. Quantitative methods collect different usability metrics and, combined with qualitative findings, mixed-methods studies offer a holistic and comprehensive understanding of the usability of HIT. The criteria with which to evaluate the quality of mixed-methods study include reliability and validity, and these quality indicators are evaluated differently in qualitative and quantitative methods. Likewise, there are different approaches to ensure the soundness and integrity of research. However, being able to demonstrate that research has been conducted in a rigorous fashion will ensure the credibility of the findings. Regardless of how many methods a researcher wants to use in conducting a mixed-methods study, feasibility is often the greatest barrier to performing complex, yet valuable mixed-methods studies, and must be considered as researchers begin to design their study.

6

Content Analysis

INTRODUCTION

This chapter provides a broad overview of how content analysis can be used to guide the discovery and analysis of qualitative data in health informatics research. Content analysis is not typically considered among the many methods used to perform user research and usability testing; however, it is an effective way to gain knowledge of the existing health messages and rhetoric embedded in HIT. The coding techniques used to analyze and sort content are used in the analysis of a broad scope of qualitative data and are applied in the data analysis of interview transcripts, survey responses, and think-aloud verbal report and observational data, which will be discussed later in the book. An exhaustive description of content analysis and coding techniques is beyond the scope of this chapter, but the primary uses of content analyses within the field of health informatics research will be discussed with a focus on three primary means of categorizing and transforming qualitative data into meaningful insight: inductive, deductive, and framework analysis. The coding techniques introduced in this chapter can be applied to analyze data collected from usability testing methods described in subsequent chapters, such as cognitive walkthroughs and think-alouds.

CONTENT ANALYSIS METHODOLOGY

Content analysis is a methodology that involves the interpretation and transformation of content into meaningful knowledge that can be used to answer

DOI: 10.1201/9781003460886-6

a wide scope of research inquiries. Historically, content analysis was termed "symbol analysis" because it developed from the scientific method of recording the number of certain keywords in mediated print publications, such as newspapers (Hamad et al., 2016). Holsti (1969) described content analysis as the application of the scientific method to identify specific characteristics of messages. Content analysis thus became a method of objectively collecting, inferring, and sorting messages into specific categories. Cartwright (1953) contended that content analysis was synonymous with coding. Given the breadth of data that is considered "content", and the depth of analysis that can be conducted, content analysis is recognized as a set of both quantitative and qualitative methods that can be applied to analyze content to yield numerical results or interpretations of the content transformed into meaningful insights (Holsti, 1969; Krippendorff, 1980).

Content, in a content analysis, is any type of textual, visual, verbal, or observational data, such as texts, websites, clinical notes, verbal transcripts, and patient education information. As such, content analysis has useful applications in the health research and HIT studies because it is an approach to exploring and describing complex phenomena related to the human experience (Elo et al., 2014; Erlingsson & Brysiewicz, 2017; Gale et al., 2013), an intimate way to engage with qualitative data, and a rich method of providing a representation of individuals' lives and HCIs situated in certain health contexts. Content analysis can be used to perform exploratory research to gain a baseline understanding of content related to HIT.

Content analysis has disciplinary roots in mass and technical communication; however, given the broad definition of what counts as "content" and its flexibility in nature, content analysis has been adopted by a number of disciplines, including nursing, library and information science, psychology, and sociology, as well as being applied by multidisciplinary teams consisting of many stakeholders: cognitive scientists, epidemiologists, health economists, management scientists, and others (Gale et al., 2013; White & Marsh, 2006). In fact, Hsiu-Fang and Shannon (2005) point out that content analysis is a popular analytic method supported by the U.S. National Institutes of Health (NIH).

Content analysis is considered a systematic and objective method of identifying and drawing inferences about content and/or messages contained in discourse by categorizing the data into themes (Hsiu-Fang et al., 2005; Krippendorff, 1980; Shuyler & Knight, 2008). Yet there are no universal rules for how to use content analysis or how the data will be categorized; therefore, it is known as a flexible method (Bengtsson, 2016; Boettger & Palmer, 2010; White et al., 2006).

Systematic Process

The systematic process for conducting a content analysis involves the following steps:

1. Identify the unit(s) of analysis.
2. Identify the sample.
3. Collect data.
4. Create coding scheme (also called a codebook) and categorize and sort data.
5. Combine or revise codes as necessary.
6. Train coders and assess reliability and validity. (This should be done concurrently with the other steps and be ongoing throughout data analysis.)

These steps will be discussed in greater detail with an example from a HIT investigation.

Qualitative Content Analysis versus Grounded Theory

Often, qualitative content analysis is confused with grounded theory; however, they are different approaches to analyzing and discussing qualitative data. The primary difference between using qualitative content analysis and grounded theory is that the purpose of a content analysis is to describe the lived experiences or phenomenon under investigation, whereby meaningful accounts or depictions are developed from the data itself (Cho & Lee, 2014; Hsiu-Fang et al., 2005). Grounded theory is aimed at developing a new theory or insight to describe a phenomenon that emerges from the data. Grounded theory is a reaction to positivism, which posits that only true knowledge can be discovered through scientific, objective methods of inquiry (Cho et al., 2014). Grounded theory is recognized as a systematic and objective method of arriving at a new theory based on qualitative comparative, iterative data analysis (Curry et al., 2009). Grounded theory does have value in qualitative research, but it involves a mutable process of reflexivity and critical inquiry that places the researcher's subjective experiences as integral to the discovery process (Bailey et al., 1999), whereas examining usability places the intended user's perspective as integral to the discovery process and the researcher's perspective as irrelevant if the end goal of qualitative research is to inform the design and delivery of usable HIT.

Consequently, grounded theory is a methodology used primarily in scholarly or academic research, when no prior knowledge or theory exists to explain the phenomenon. It has limited practical applications in HIT usability research, which aims to obtain useful findings that can be used to improve the usability of HIT. That said, grounded theory has been paired with other analytical techniques within the same study. Alpert et al. (2017) used grounded theory to inductively develop codes that grouped interview and focus group transcript data, then used a more focused approach to deductively sort the results into predetermined codes established by the uses and gratifications (U&G) framework. Grounded theory will not be discussed further in this book, but I wanted to call attention to the methodology to avoid confusion in coding techniques.

Identify the Unit(s) of Analysis

As discussed in Chapter 5, your research questions should drive the design of your study. For instance, if you want to understand the usability of a clinical decision support system (CDSS) that uses the Framingham Assessment to aggregate patient medical data and make predictions regarding the patient's risk of coronary heart disease from the clinician's perspective, you will first need to identify how you will measure usability (clinician's sentiment when interacting with the system, time on task, task success rate, etc.), and be prepared to recruit a sample population of representative users (physicians who would likely use the CDSS in practice) to be the subjects in your study.

Similarly, a content analysis is informed by your research questions. The unit(s) of analysis is/are the content that constitutes the data you collect to analyze. Content can be any type of communication or discourse, of any form, that conveys meaning from a sender to a receiver (Shannon & Weaver, 1998). A wide variety of textual, visual, and user interface content can be collected as data to analyze (Hsiu-Fang et al., 2005). Below are some categories of type of content and units of analysis that correspond with each type.

- *Textual.* Written health information; interview transcripts; field notes; verbal report transcriptions; publications/literature; diaries; physician and patient communications; job advertisements; emails; letters; SOAP notes; etc.
- *Visual.* Images; figures; pictures; observational records on video; films; videos; web pages, etc.
- *User interface.* Icons, buttons, color scheme, layout, font size, etc.

Verbal content from interviews or focus group discussion is generally audio-recorded and must be transcribed verbatim to be used as content analysis data.

Often, when investigating HIT, a mixture of content is collected as data. Images and textual data are subject to analysis if a researcher is investigating a health information website. Likewise, the user interface elements with which an individual interacts, such as the buttons, navigation menu, and chat box, as well as the text on a mHealth application, could be collected and coded simultaneously in a content analysis.

Identify the Sample

A sample of content is a smaller, manageable set of texts, interfaces, or other communications that you will analyze as the content in your study. Your research aim and environment should drive the determination of your content sample (Cavanagh, 1997). Samples must be selected to ensure the inclusion of relevant features, ideas, messages, and other elements associated with the phenomenon under investigation. Developing a systematic method to select a sample of content allows researchers to ensure that their sample is reflective of the wider corpus of data that is relevant to their phenomenon under investigation and that the sample content will be able to be analyzed ways that offer valuable implications for your research inquiry, which is to say that you are able to answer your research question(s). For instance, if your research aim is to understand patients' perceptions of telemedicine visits, then you will likely collect qualitative data, such as interviews with patients, clinician notes, and possibly SMS messages to patients. A representative sample should be collected from the patients and clinicians relevant to your research inquiry. Are you interested in examining telemedicine visits that occur in certain states, in certain communities, and/or by certain demographics? Answers to these types of questions will be unique for every individual study; however, your sample content must be representative of the subject being studied (Cavanagh, 1997).

The larger the sample size, the greater the generalizability of the findings; however, there is no standard formula for determining sample size. It often depends on time and resources available to conduct the study.

In my examination of direct-to-consumer telemedicine websites, I wanted to understand what rhetorical messages and information existing DTC telemedicine providers provisioned on their consumer-facing websites and be able to compare larger telemedicine providers that have more resources with smaller, less-experienced telemedicine providers (Campbell, 2020b). The content I was analyzing was DTC telemedicine websites, and I narrowed down my sample population to three DTC telemedicine providers: Teladoc, KADAN Institute, and Carie Health (Campbell, 2020b). This sample allowed me to analyze the content and draw comparisons in ways that addressed one of my primary research inquiries.

Petch (2004) performed a similar content analysis, aiming to understand the various interests of health information producers who delivered health information online, and to evaluate the quality of the information disseminated online by those health information producers. Considering that there are numerous health information providers that disseminate health information through a variety of channels, such as social media platforms, radio, television, kiosks, interpersonal communication with healthcare professionals, and more, Petch (2004) performed a systematic process of selecting the sample of health information websites (the unit of analysis) to analyze, which was guided by the primary research inquiry. To compare different health information producers' purposes for maintaining a health information website, Petch (2004) selected to analyze the websites of three different sectors of organizations that delivered health information online: government, non-profit, and commercial. From this large data corpus, Petch (2004, p. 20) sampled seven websites to analyze:

> The websites chosen from the government sector were pre-determined by the field supervisors and were selected to complement their own current research interests. The research selected the website form the non-profit and commercial sector. The criteria for including in this study required that the website be 1) written in English, and, 2) non-topic specific (i.e. offer general health information to one or more groups).

The important point about selecting your sample is that the process must be able to be reproduced or replicated if another researcher were to repeat your study or conduct a similar study. Therefore, you must document the steps you took to select your sample and clearly describe your sampling method in the methods section when you publish your research.

Collect Data

Next, collect your data. Once you have decided on a unit of analysis and sample, you can begin to collect the data. Given that content analysis can be used on a broad scope of what "counts" as content, and that there are no specific rules that must be followed when collecting the data, how best to collect and manage the content to be analyzed is the researcher's decision.

Researchers can use different tools and techniques to collect data depending on the type of content collected. There are many qualitative data analysis software (QDAS) products that can be used to aggregate content to be analyzed by individuals or multidisciplinary teams. Top QDAS products include NVivo (qsrinternational.com/nvivo-qualitative-data-analysis-software/home), ATLAS. ti (atlasti.com), and MAXQDA (maxqda.com). QDAS offer many affordances:

- Easy upload of qualitative data
- Ease and thoroughness with data management
- Integration with many qualitative data collection instruments, such as survey tools
- Efficiency
- Multiple media files uploads
- Flexibility in coding
- Collaboration on multidisciplinary teams
- Increased thoroughness and handling of data management
- Statistical analysis
- Export of visualizations.

Depending on the type of content you are analyzing, different QDAS may be more suited to handle that particular qualitative data. For instance, QSR International's NVivo 12 qualitative data analysis software can store and manage media files, such as audio and video recordings uploaded as mp3 and mp4 files. NVivo allows for the coding of video and audio recordings as one unit (the verbal reports are able to be depicted and coded in the context of the interaction). This allows for a more enriching, more intimate interaction with content, which allows for better or more accurate inferences to be made. When selecting a QDSA, it is important that it is suitable for the content that you are analyzing and will support the tasks you need to perform to analyze the data.

Often, a simple spreadsheet will do, and can be used effectively to conduct a content analysis. When the purpose is to perform word counts or gain an understanding of the presence of certain words, a QDAS may be the appropriate route to go to be able to quickly perform word frequencies and statistical analyses; however, when collecting data where the units are less clear, such as a user interface or website, which can vary in size, structure, and the presentation of textual and visual information, using a spreadsheet may be more suitable to be able to collect content in meaningful ways according to a framework you either emulate from another study or develop specifically for your study.

When collecting textual data, you may transcribe audio-recorded interviews and aggregate all your data into one document. If you are collecting survey responses, you may be able to export survey results as a spreadsheet or upload directly into a QDAS. Or, when collecting a sample of user interface content or website content, a plus (+)/minus (−) technique can be applied, whereby you are guided by predefined criteria and each interface is assigned a plus (+) if it appears to exhibit any level of detail defined by the guidance criteria for each code and a minus (−) if it does not provide any content or reference to the information defined by the guidance criteria for each code. Table 6.1 illustrates the set-up of a spreadsheet that was used to analyze telemedicine websites using the plus (+)/minus (−) technique.

The plus (+)/minus (−) technique involves the simultaneous process of coding; however, when collecting data, you will want to make note of quotes, responses, or passages of text; capture screen shots; collect images, pictures, and/or other content that are representative of the particular phenomenon under investigation to use in the results or discussion section when you publish your research (Campbell, 2020b). These might be examples you use to illustrate a code or as evidence to corroborate your inferences. The plus (+)/minus (−) technique may also be used when performing a sentiment analysis, whereby the emotional reaction or affective state of a human subject is evaluated or inferred from qualitative data. In a sentiment analysis, a plus (+) may be used next to text to indicate a positive emotional reaction and a minus (−) may be used to indicate the subject had a negative reaction to a particular stimulus or interaction with technology.

Create Coding Scheme (Also Called a Codebook) and Categorize and Sort Data

Creating a coding scheme or codebook may be the most challenging, yet most insightful, part of conducting a content analysis. Coding involves the sorting of content into categories of related content or themes that have similar meaning. These condensed meaning units are provided a descriptive label and called "codes." Content can be condensed and further subdivided into smaller units under main codes, which are termed "subcodes." The purpose of creating a codebook is to provide a means to describe the phenomenon under investigation, increase understanding, and generate knowledge (Cavanagh, 1997).

The coding of qualitative data supports HIT usability research by generating a deep and nuanced understanding of the HIT under investigation and providing a detailed description of the content and its relationship with HIT usability. Coding allows researchers to identify patterns in data. Simply put, developing conceptual categories or themes to sort content brings meaning to the data set. There are several approaches to coding content. Three effective

TABLE 6.1

Using a spreadsheet to perform data analysis using the plus (+)/minus (–) technique

Code/theme	Criteria	Yes (+)	No (–)
Knowledge	Information about the service (what it is and how to use it).	Yes (+)	
Outcomes	Noting what will be done with the results. Identification that the patient will be diagnosed and prescribed medications if needed.	Yes (+)	
Reassurance	Technology and equipment are easy to use (reassurance to patients they do not need to have high technical literacy). Noting patients have support for technical problems.	Yes (+)	
Benefits	Confidentiality is ensured. Cost is low. Noting the benefits to users.	Yes (+)	
Choice	Noting that the service is optional and not a substitute for traditional face-to-face physician consultations. Noting that the service is not a substitute for emergency services.	Yes (+)	
Previous experience	Testimonials: patients' quotes about positive use of service to encourage potential consumers to use it. Identification of who to contact for further information.		No (–)
Further information	Identification of who will help the patient if they need help.	Yes (+)	
Appearance	Visuals, images, and graphics are included. Information visuals are used as an alternative means of providing information to users. Diversity (age, ethnicity, gender) is used in visuals.	Yes (+)	

Source: Campbell (2020b).

and commonly used coding methods in health communication literature are inductive, deductive, and framework analysis. Both inductive and deductive coding are types of thematic analysis, but reside on opposite ends of the thematic analysis continuum. The major distinction between these two approaches is that inductive coding has the researcher generate themes or codes that arise during data analysis, whereas deductive coding, or direct coding, uses an a priori codebook or a pre-existing coding scheme that guides the researcher in sorting content into categories.

Conventional Content Analysis Using an Inductive Approach

In a conventional content analysis, researchers allow the themes or categories of related content emerge from the data (Hsiu-Fang et al., 2005). There is no coding scheme (codes previously identified in literature) that a researcher has to guide them to sort the content into similarly-related meaning units; rather, they use their own interpretation of the data to make inferences or best-guess choices about how to sort the content and label codes. Inductive coding relies heavily on the researcher's expertise regarding the subject matter, context of the study, and creativity in creating descriptive code names (Bailey et al., 1999; Elo et al., 2014). Inductive coding is an iterative process whereby researchers sort and sift through data to identify similar meanings or relationships, continuously compare categories and constructs with the content, and revisit content and codes as new codes emerge during data analysis.

Chew and Eysenbach (2010) performed a content analysis of a sample of Twitter posts to monitor the use of pandemic-related terms and the public's attention to and sentiment toward these posts. Chew et al. (2010) used an inductive approach to reflect on the Tweet's content, how it was expressed, and the link posted to develop preliminary codes, then after collaborative review of the codes, collapsed infrequently used codes into larger concepts that resulted in the development of a final codebook sorting content into categories such as Resource, Personal Experience, and Marketing. Table 6.2 shows Chew et al.'s (2010) codebook.

Codebooks or coding schemes, like Chew et al.'s (2010) in Table 6.2, often include the following columns of information: code, subcodes (if applicable), description, and example. Including these various pieces of information lends a hand in increasing the transferability, replicability, and reliability of the content analysis because it provides specific, concrete details for when a code should be applied to a particular piece of content that can be used by researchers in relevant studies. A useful codebook might just include the primary code and directions for when to apply the code to qualitative data, such as Kushniruk & Borycki's (2015) codebook developed for the analysis of empirical data obtained from usability testing with human subjects (see Table 6.3).

Developing a codebook that can be easily applied by multidisciplinary teams and in future research supports the development of knowledge and insight that enhances HIT usability and encourages collaboration among multiple stakeholders invested in a study. Furthermore, having clear criteria for how to apply a code supports the training that may be required when hiring coders.

TABLE 6.2

Descriptions and examples of content categories from the content analysis of pandemic-related tweets

Content	Description	Example tweets
Resource	Tweet contains H1N1 news, updates, or information. May be the title or summary of the linked article. Contents may or may not be factual.	*"China Reports First Case of Swine Flu (New York Times): A 30-year-old man who flew from St. Louis to Chengdu is ... " http://tinyurl.com/rdbhcg* *"Ways to Prevent Flu" http://tinyurl.com/r4/4cx#swineflu#h1n1"*
Personal experience	Twitter user mentions a direct (personal) or indirect (e.g., friend, family, co-worker) experience with the H1N1 virus or the social/economic effects of H1N1.	*"Swine flu panic almost stopped me from going to US, but now back from my trip and so happy I went :-))"* *"Oh we got a swine flu leaflet. clearly the highlight of my day"* *"My sister has swine flu!"*
Personal opinion and Interest	Twitter user posts their opinion of the H1N1 virus/situation/news or expresses a need for or discovery of information. General H1N1 chatter or commentary.	*"More people have died from normal flu than swine flu, it's just a media hoax, to take people's mind off the recession"* *"Currently looking up some info on H1N1"* *"Swine flu is scary!"*
Jokes/parody	Tweet contains a H1N1 joke told via video, text, or photo; or a humorous opinion of H1N1 that does not refer to a personal experience.	*"If you're an expert on the swine flu, does that make you fluent?"*
Marketing	Tweet contains an advertisement for an H1N1-related product or service.	*"Buy liquid vitamin C as featured in my video" http://is.gd/y87r#health#hin1"*
Spam	Tweet is unrelated to H1N1.	*"musicmonday MM lamarodom Yom Kippur Polanski Jay-Z H1N1 Watch FREE online LATEST MOVIES at http://a.gd/b1586f"*

Source: Chew and Eysebach et al. (2010).

Directed Content Analysis Using a Deductive Approach

In a directed content analysis, the researcher uses a pre-existing coding scheme during data analysis. A directed content analysis is more structured than a conventional approach because the codes the research will use to sort and categorize data

TABLE 6.3

Coding categories for identifying surface-level usability issues in HIT

Video code	When applied
Navigation	Coded when a review of the video data indicates that the user has problems moving through a system or user interface.
Consistency	Coded when a review of the video indicates that the user has problems due to a lack of consistency in the user interface.
Meaning of icons/terminology	Coded when a review of the video data indicates that the user does not understand language or labels used in the interface.
Visibility of system status	Coded when a review of the video data indicates that the user does not know what the system is doing.
Understanding error messages	Coded when a review of the video data indicates that the user does not understand meaning of error messages.
Understanding instructions	Coded when a review of the video data indicates that the user does not understand user instructions.
Workflow issues	Coded when a review of the video data indicates that there are issues with system workflow negatively impacting user interaction.
Graphics	Coded when a review of the video data indicates that there are issues with graphics.
Layout	Coded when a review of the video data indicates that there are problems with the layout of screens or information on those screens.
Speed/response time	Coded when a review of the video data indicates that the system is slow or response time is an issue.
Color	Coded when a review of the video data indicates that the user does not like the color or color schemes used in the interface.
Font	Coded when a review of the video data indicates that the font is too small or not readable.
Overall ease of use	Coded when the user comments on overall usability of the user interface.

Source: Kushniruk et al. (2015).

have already been identified in the literature; the researcher reviews the content to identify all instances of content that correspond with or exemplify any of the pre-identified categories (Hsiu-Fang et al., 2005). For novice qualitative researchers, using a deductive approach may be easier and less intimidating because they can start with an a priori codebook, which eliminates the need to create labels or determine the initial coding scheme that will be used to describe the phenomenon under investigation. When using an a priori coding scheme, it is important to use one that relates to a similar HIT under investigation or aims to identify the same type of features or aspects of the phenomenon you are investigating; otherwise, the findings will not help you answer your research questions.

I used an a priori codebook developed by Kayyali et al. (2017) in my content analysis of telemedicine provider websites (Campbell, 2020b). Because Kayyali et al.'s (2017) study provided a coding scheme that included the criteria by which I wanted to evaluate the telemedicine providers, such as rhetorical messages and use of visuals, it afforded me a useful and relevant codebook to use for my content analysis. Additionally, Kayyali et al.'s (2017) study investigated similar health information media and had similar research inquiries; thus their codebook had valuable implications for my study. I used a directed approach and Kayyali et al.'s (2017) codebook (see Table 6.4) to code the content displayed and delivered on telemedicine provider websites.

TABLE 6.4

Rhetorical/content code and guidance criteria used for analysis of telemedicine provider websites

Code/theme	Guidance criteria
Outcomes	• Noting what will be done with the results. • Identification that the patient will be diagnosed and prescribed medications if needed.
Reassurance	• Technology and equipment is easy to use (reassurance to patients they do not need to have high technical literacy). • Noting patients have support for technical problems. • Confidentiality is ensured. • Cost is low.
Benefits	• Noting the benefits to users.
Choice	• Noting the service is optional and not a substitute for traditional face-to-face physician consultations. • Noting that the service is not a substitute for emergency services.
Previous experience	• Testimonials. • Patients' quotes about positive use of service to encourage potential consumers to use it.
Further information	• Identification of who to contact for further information. • Identification of who will help the patient if they need help.
Appearance	• Visuals, images, and graphics are included. • Information visuals are used as an alternative means of providing information to users. • Diversity (age, ethnicity, gender) is used in visuals.
Readability	• Readability of health information (text) compared with recommended sixth grade level. • Use of Flesch-Kincaid Grade Level (FKGL).

Source: Campbell (2020b); adapted from Kayyali et al. (2017).

This approach allowed me to systematically order and sort the content available on the telemedicine provider websites into the types of information they provide to the user and the extent to which they guide users to performing a virtual doctor visit. It should be noted that Kayyali et al. (2017) used an *inductive* approach to coding in their content analysis of telemedicine leaflets. After reviewing the literature, it was determined that the only relevant existing codebook lacked some of the criteria by which they wanted to evaluate the leaflets for, thus they inductively developed the coding scheme that I then used for my study. This is an example of how one study can result in the development of a coding scheme that can be used in future research that contributes to the body of knowledge on the subject matter.

In another example, Khajouei et al. (2017) used predetermined codes to identify and categorize usability problems that were discovered during two different usability inspection methods: heuristic evaluation and cognitive walkthrough. Aiming to compare the number and severity of usability problems identified when using each method, Khajouei et al. (2017) used an a priori codebook including the usability attributes synthesized from Nielsen (1993a) and the ISO's (2018) usability models to categorize each usability problem that was identified in each of the methods. After collecting the data, consisting of usability problems, Khajouel et al. (2017) sorted each data point according to the usability attribute to which it failed to adhere: effectiveness, efficiency, satisfaction, learnability, memorability, and errors. To compare different data sets, it is best to use the same coding procedure and codebook. This also provides a means to triangulate data because each data set was analyzed and interpreted in the same way.

Despite using a directed approach, data that cannot be coded under a predetermined category within the initial coding scheme should be given a new code. The goal of qualitative research is to be able to describe and discover new understandings of a particular phenomenon; therefore, if you discover emergent themes that do not fit under an existing theme, it would be advisable to add this code to your codebook. The purpose of a directed content analysis is to test an existing theory or extend prior knowledge by examining content and sorting it into the existing categories; however, by ignoring or neglecting to account for data that do not fit under a predetermined category, you may not capture new insights about the phenomenon under investigation or be able to articulate your new discovery. As emerging areas related the phenomenon of interest and the HIT under investigation are identified, they need to be included when analyzing content in order to improve and broaden the frameworks used to evaluate HIT (Kushniruk et al., 2019a). This leads to the last coding technique discussed that is relevant to health information content analysis and coding of qualitative data.

Framework Analysis: Blending Inductive and Deductive Coding

Framework analysis has significant implications for health research because of the affordances it offers multidisciplinary teams in analyzing data. Framework analysis is another thematic analysis technique. During the application of framework analysis, as the name applies, a matrix is formed of rows (cases), columns (codes), and cells structuring the data so it can be explored as individual units (one interviewee's response) or comparatively across the data corpus (all interviewees' responses) (Ritchie & Lewis, 2003). Framework analysis can be conducted using a combination of inductive and deductive approaches. Although the systematic "constant comparative" method used to search for common themes and patterns across qualitative data is associated with grounded theory, framework analysis differentiates itself by the primary objective for using the technique is to discover relationships and common themes related to the phenomenon of interest in order to provide a comprehensive descriptive account of the phenomenon, whereas grounded theory is concerned with developing new social theory (Gale et al., 2013). Framework analysis is a time-intensive, task-intensive technique that is best-suited for QDAS.

Framework analysis is a coding technique typically applied to interview and focus group transcript data consisting of five main steps allowing researchers to intimately acquaint themselves with the data and make inferences based on their own unique perspective (Srivastava & Thomson, 2009):

Step 1: Familiarize. The researchers immerse themselves in the data to familiarize themselves with the content. Researchers may re-listen to interview audio recordings and reread interview transcripts.

Step 2: Identify a thematic framework. After becoming familiar with the qualitative data, researchers identify common themes or emerging issues associated with the phenomenon of interest. Themes represent semantic topics and must arise from the data and be newly classified or they can be recognized from previously established frameworks. Both inductive and deductive analysis can be used when developing and refining a thematic framework. It involves both logical and intuitive thinking because it requires the researcher to make inferences about the meaning and importance of issues, as well as implicit connections between ideas (Srivastava et al., 2009). When working on a multidisciplinary team, it is important to be open, critical, and reflexive when creating the thematic framework to account for multiple perspectives.

Step 3: Index. Next, after a thematic framework has been agreed upon by all multidisciplinary team members, the data corpus is coded according to the thematic framework. This generally involves going line by line and applying numbers that represent each theme according to the thematic framework. Using an ordinal system allows anomalies in the data to recognized and reconciled between researchers, which increases the richness of the analysis (Gale et al., 2013).

Step 4: Chart. The matrix is formed in the fourth stage, which involves transferring the ordinal system and associated content to a matrix consisting of headings, subheadings, and the pieces of content coded in each of the categories. It is important that the content is still associated with the individual case from which it originated—for example, from each individual interviewee. Forming this matrix allows patterns to emerge among particular individuals or all individuals, which help illuminate the phenomenon under investigation. It is important to condense data enough to fit into the matrix, yet also retain the original meanings and tone of the subject's verbalization. Illustrative quotes and other annotations should also be included in the matrix; annotations can be included in the margin beside the text or tagged automatically if you use a QDAS. It is recommended that cases be kept in the same order in each chart (Ritchie & Spencer, 1994).

Step 5: Map and interpret. The final step involves analyzing and interpretating key characteristics that are illustrated by the matrix. The process of analysis and interpretation can include:

- identifying similar and different characteristics between cases
- generating typologies
- interrogating theoretical concepts
- identifying usability problems
- exploring relationships and/or causality
- creating descriptive accounts
- making predictions about user responses
- developing strategies (Gale et al., 2013; Srivastava et al., 2009).

Framework analysis is an effective coding technique by which to explore qualitative data, which is often the type of data that is gathered during usability testing. It is systematic and provides an audit trail, therefore qualifying as a rigorous approach to qualitative data analysis. Yet framework analysis is fluid enough to be ideally used by multidisciplinary teams because it requires critical reflexivity and open-mindedness to multiple interpretations. Framework analysis affords a comprehensive and holistic understanding of the phenomenon of interest. Although task intensive, the matrix that is formed during data analysis reduces and structures data in a useful visual layout that facilitates deep engagement and the recognition of patterns across a corpus of data (Gale et al., 2013; Srivastava et al., 2009).

> The unique aspects of "framework" are (a) the matrix which is very valuable for undertaking constant comparative analysis across themes and across cases and (b) the summaries of data that go in the cells of the matrix. In my view, this summarization process is a really valuable thing to do for two reasons: (i) it forces the analyst to think carefully about the essence of what the respondent has said, rather than trying to interpret too quickly and (ii) it allows other members of the interdisciplinary teams (non-qual specialists) to engage with the data meaningfully without having to read all the transcripts, so it can enhance reflexivity and interdisciplinary thinking.
> (N. K. Gale, personal communication, August 16, 2021)

It should be noted that framework analysis should not be used by novice researchers who are unfamiliar with the approach. It may require training and researchers need to be able to think creatively and creatively to inductively code content (Bailey et al., 1999; Gale et al., 2013).

To explicate how to perform each of the steps in framework analysis, Zolnoori et al.'s (2019) study will be used. A multidisciplinary team used framework analysis when conducting a content analysis of patient-generated content on health forums. The purpose of Zolnoori et al.'s (2019) study was to gain a comprehensive understanding of the factors affecting patients' attitudes toward antidepressants and the disease-management strategies used for patients with diabetes who also had financial difficulties. As mentioned in Chapter 5, one's research questions should drive the study design and selection of data collection instruments and analysis techniques. Cultivating a broad understanding of these unique subjective and contextual factors affecting healthcare is a primary focus of heath research; thus, framework analysis was selected as the qualitative content analysis technique because it is best suited to achieve this aim. Zolnoori et al. (2019) state that, "This process can provide deep insight into textual data for identifying patterns and various aspects of textual content."

Subsequent to collecting a sample of representative textual content from health forums discussing patients' experience with the healthcare system using text mining tools (MetaMap or Text Analysis and Knowledge Extraction System), Zolnoori et al. (2019) performed the first step in framework analysis: familiarizing themselves with the data. Zolnoori et al. (2019) analyzed the content and established that the unit of analysis would be a sentence from patients' comments because it had to be large enough to convey a perspective and small enough to be kept as a meaningful unit of analysis.

Next, Zolnoori et al. (2019) used previously established themes discovered in their literature review that were useful for summarizing patient experiences with antidepressants in online forums. Their thematic framework consisted of five main themes. For each theme, they developed an operational definition that offered clear guidance for coding purposes (see Table 6.5), similar to Chew et al.

TABLE 6.5

Predefined thematic framework for identifying patients' experiences with antidepressants and operational definitions of each theme

Categories	Factors (predefined codes)	Description
Pharmacological treatment factors	Perceived effectiveness	The patient's subjective assessment of antidepressant helpfulness in the reduction of depression symptoms, enhancing emotional and cognitive functionalities, and overall enhancement of quality of life.
	Perceived necessity	The patient's subjective assessment of antidepressant necessity in improving and maintaining current and future health conditions. For example, the patient may find an antidepressant vital in reducing the risk of relapse.
	Perceived concern	The patient's subjective assessment of harmful effects of antidepressants in the long term. The patient may view antidepressants as addictive, taking control over feelings and thoughts, and altering personality in the long term.
	Side-effects	Any adverse reactions to antidepressants intake that the patient reports. Antidepressants' adverse reactions may include physiological side-effects, emotional syndromes, cognitive impairment, and limitations on daily functioning, and overall reduction in quality of life.
	Perceived distress from side-effects	The patient's perceived distress from antidepressants side-effects depends on the patient's self-attention to the internal bodily sensations that may have an influence on patient tolerability of side-effects. The patient may show distress by using adjectives showing severity of the side-effects, negative impact on work or daily activities, or visiting the emergency department. A severe side-effect, including self-harm and suicidal ideation or attempt, also reflects high perceived distress.
Healthcare system factors	Patient–provider relationship	The patient expresses their satisfaction or dissatisfaction with healthcare providers from various aspects, such as perceived support from providers or perception of healthcare providers' knowledge about illness and treatment.
	Healthcare settings	The patient may demonstrate a higher level of trust and satisfaction towards diagnosis and treatment offered in a psychiatric setting compared with a primary care setting.
	Affordability	The patient may complain about the high cost of antidepressants and the lack of insurance coverage.

TABLE 6.5 (Continued)

Predefined thematic framework for identifying patients' experiences with antidepressants and operational definitions of each theme

Categories	Factors (predefined codes)	Description
Psycho-social factors	Stigma and cultural related factors	The patient may express their concerns about stigma and cultural-related factors that may make the prolonged pharmacological treatment notoriously difficult for patients. For example, the public may view antidepressant intake as a sign of weakness or incapacity to deal with daily emotional distress that may influence patient acceptance of antidepressants.
	Partner support	The patient may express their perceived support from partners (family and friends) about having depression as proper diagnosis and having an antidepressant as a proper treatment.
Patient- related factors	General concern and necessity	The patient may express their general view towards medications. For example, they may view all medications as harmful and believe natural remedies and changing lifestyle will have a better healthcare outcome than pharmacological treatment.

Source: Zolnoori et al. (2019).

(2010) (see Table 6.2), Kushniruk et al. (2015) (see Table 6.3), and Campbell (2020b) (see Table 6.4).

When indexing the content, Zolnoori et al. (2019) performed both deductive and inductive analysis by coding content according to the previously established framework and generating new themes when content did not fit into the existing framework. The constant comparative method, consistent with open coding, and the development of operational definitions for each predefined theme and emergent themes allow the multidisciplinary team to uniformly code the sample of content. The final codebook developed from the study illustrates different dimensions and aspects of patients' experiences and can also be used to test hypotheses concerning the relationships between the variables that affect patients' experiences in the healthcare system (Zolnoori et al., 2019).

To structure the data into the matrix, the coding environment selected was a spreadsheet, which allowed for the data to be entered into columns and rows. Codes typically run along the top as columns, and each individual point of case data is entered in a row allowing for analysis of an individual case, an individual theme, or across the entire data corpus (see Table 6.6).

TABLE 6.6

Sentences from patient posts (unit of analysis) organized in the rows and themes (adverse drug reactions) organized in the columns

comment_Id	drug_Id	sentence index	sentences	ADR	WD	EF	INF	PPI-P	PPI-N	KN	SS	ADR-PA	ADR-NA	WD-PA	WD-NA	Others
1	EffexorXR.1	1	Total nightmare.										1			
1	EffexorXR.1	2	This was arguably the worst period of time in my life.										1			1
1	EffexorXR.1	3	It made me so mentally ill I almost ended up in a psych ward.	1												
1	EffexorXR.1	4	Stay away from this if you can!													
1	EffexorXR.1	5	I lost weight considerably and shook all the time.	1												
1	EffexorXR.1	6	I had terrible anxiety the whole time, the worst kind of anxiety I've ever experienced.	1			1						1			
1	EffexorXR.1	7	Also tardive diskenesia was becoming very prevalent.	1												
1	EffexorXR.1	8	Tabacco cravings were rampant.	1												
1	EffexorXR.1	9	I never felt at ease or comfortable, I was constantly on edge and wanted to cry.	1												
1	EffexorXR.1	10	Please be careful if you are taking this, o	1												1

2	EffexorXR.2	1	Sleepy, constipated, unable to orgasm, felt "out of body" most of the time.	1			
2	EffexorXR.2	2	Some improvement in mood but not worth it, at all	1		1	
2	EffexorXR.2	3	Withdrawal is difficult and unpleasant.	1		1	
2	EffexorXR.2	4	Would not recommend this drug to anyone.	1			1
3	EffexorXR.3	1	Extreme irritability, weight gain and sleepless are just a few side effects of this horrible drug.	1	1	1	
3	EffexorXR.3	2	Sure it helps depression because it makes you not give a rats ass about anything!	1	1		
3	EffexorXR.3	3	I was on 225 mg and have weaned down to 37,5.	1			
3	EffexorXR.3	4	The only way I can sum it up is to say I wish I could be put to sleep for a month or so while this gets out of my system.	1		1	
3	EffexorXR.3	5	Horrible Horrible Horrible	1			1
4	EffexorXR.4	1	I tried to kill myself witch mad no sense since I LOVE MY LIFE!	1			1

(Continued)

TABLE 6.6 (Continued)

Sentences from patient posts (unit of analysis) organized in the rows and themes (adverse drug reactions) organized in the columns

comment_Id	drug_Id	sentence index	sentences	ADR	WD	EF	INF	PPI-P	PPI-N	KN	SS	ADR-PA	ADR-NA	WD-PA	WD-NA	Others
4	EffexorXR.4	2	The effexor worked great at first and then slowly i started to sleep more and feel more and more depressed, I also started having weird behavior.	1	1	1	1									
4	EffexorXR.4	3	I never tried to hurt myself before this drug, o	1			1									
5	EffexorXR.5	1	Constipation, drastic mood swings, 100% helped my anxiety and panic.	1		1		1								
5	EffexorXR.5	2	didn't do much for the depression.				1									
5	EffexorXR.5	3	This drug is the devil.									1				
5	EffexorXR.5	4	Ever try getting off of it?													
5	EffexorXR.5	5	You would think you were going through heroin withdrawals.											1		
5	EffexorXR.5	6	Im lucky I didn't die b/c I just stopped cold turkey one day and the brain zaps puking and overall feeling you get is like no other.	1												1

5	EffexorXR.5	7	I will never touch an antidepressant again.		1
5	EffexorXR.5	8	Just to think that I went through all that physical and mental anguish to get off a drug.	1	1
5	EffexorXR.5	9	it could not be safe to take on a daily basis.		1

Note: Each case assigned a value of "1" indicates the theme to which that content was assigned in the thematic framework. Themes are abbreviated—for example, ADR = adverse drug reaction; WD = withdrawal symptoms; EF = effectiveness. (Zolnoori et al. (2019).

Finally, in the last step, Zolnoori et al. (2019) leveraged the highly structured data to make interpretations and draw conclusions regarding the identified patterns and trends they discovered in the process of analyzing the content.

> The matrix structure provides an intuitively structured overview of the summarized data that can facilitate and accelerate the identification of patterns and themes by highlighting the contradictory data and irregular cases. More importantly, it keeps a clear map between original data and themes in the analytical framework, indicating illustrative quotes for themes.
>
> (Zolnoori et al., 2019)

Framework analysis is an effective and useful approach to content analysis because it blends deductive analysis, which is informed by previous relevant research, and inductive analysis, which allows for new insight to emerge from a deep exploration of qualitative data. Research questions drive study designs, data collection instruments, and data analysis tools and techniques. Zolnoori et al. (2019) were able to achieve their primary aims for the investigation of patients' experiences in the healthcare system gleaned from their comments posted on health forums by identifying the underlying factors associated with patients' attitudes toward antidepressants.

Summative Content Analysis

Hsiu-Fang et al. (2005) describe a third coding technique, summative analysis, whereby specific keywords are searched for in relation to particular content and the researcher makes interpretations of the contextual meaning of these instances and how it applies to or affects the phenomenon under investigation. In this way, summative content analysis includes both quantitative and qualitive methods by first analyzing specific word frequencies, then focusing on discovering the underlying meaning of these words within the context or exploring for the appearance of similar terms and making inferences of their usages.

Combine or Revise Codes as Necessary

As you continue to perform data analysis and sort content into the appropriate categories, you may find that there are infrequently used codes or very similar themes of content that you can combine into one main theme or code. Depending on the level of abstraction that you perform, you may also develop subcodes, whereby the main themes are simply larger meaning units that are abstracted into subthemes. Themes or codes represent semantic topics but may be further refined into subthemes related to the main theme. For instance,

TABLE 6.7

Telemedicine interface usability themes, subcodes, and descriptions

Usability Dimension/Code	Subcode	Description
Screens	Home Screens	Have a simple and engaging home screen.
	Registration	Make registration and logging in as simple and obvious as possible.
Content	Hierarchy	Put the most important information first.
	Positive Tone	Stay positive and realistic. Include the benefits of taking action.
	Specific	Provide specific action steps.
	Spacious	Display content clearly on the page.
	*Cost/Pricing	Clearly display the cost or fees for a virtual physician visit or clearly identify common health insurance plan costs for the benefit.
	*Restricted Access	Do not require one to log in or create an account to find out more information about membership or benefits.
	*Privacy, Confidentiality, and Security	Make evident that individuals' personal information remains private and confidential, and that transfer of data is secure.
	*Updated/Relevant Content	Provide frequent updates to content that are relevant and current.
Display	Font	Ensure the font is easy to read.
	Contrast	Use bold colors with contrast and avoid dark or busy backgrounds.
	Accessibility	Make the system accessible to people with disabilities.
Navigation	Topics	Put topics in multiple categories.
	Orientation	Enable easy access to home and menu screens.
	Back Button	Make sure the "Back" button works.
	Linear Navigation	Use linear information paths (e.g., numbered screens).
	Buttons	Simplify screen-based controls and enlarged buttons.
	Links	Label links clearly and use them effectively.
	Search	Include simple search and browse options.
	*Mobile Responsiveness	Design content to be mobile-responsiveness and important information easy to find on mobile devices.
Interactivity	Multimedia	Incorporate audio and visual features.
	New Media	Explore new media such as Twitter or text messaging
*Performance	*Page Loading Speed	Support fast loading of website and individual webpages.
*No Usability Improvements Required	*Easy to Use or Intuitive	Interface is user-friendly and designed to make information intuitively easy to find.

Source: Adapted from HHS (n.d.) and Monkman et al. (2013a) (*Newly added emergent codes identified during data analysis) (Campbell, 2020b; Campbell et al., 2022).

when analyzing representative user-generated responses regarding how to improve the usability of a telemedicine website, my colleague and I used an a priori codebook consisting of main codes and subcodes to code respondents' subjective comments, but as new semantics emerged that were not able to be categorized under an existing code in the codebook, new codes and subcodes were developed and provided an operational definition, thereby expanding on the codebook (Campbell, 2020b; Campbell & Monkman, 2022).

The final codebook or coding scheme developed should have a sufficient level of construct validity. Construct validity is difficult to appraise when analyzing qualitative data; construct validity is the extent to which a code or theme accurately represents or measures the concept being assessed (White et al., 2006). The difficulty lies in the fact that often inferences from qualitative data made by researchers are subjective and inherently biased because every researcher has a unique personal and scholarly history and subscribes to different scientific paradigms that may shape their perspective. Additionally, Stemler (2001) says to be conscientious of the individuals who have been developing the coding scheme have often been so intimately fixated on the data and project that they may have established shared and hidden meanings of the coding scheme, which is another reason why establishing a clear codebook is so valuable. One way to establish a high level of construct validity is to develop a coding scheme with clear operational definitions, instructions for when to apply a code, and unambiguous examples taken directly from the content. All these features increase the likelihood that all coders will code the same item the same way or that a coder will code the same item the same way at different points in time (White et al., 2006). Additionally, if the coding scheme is modified during the data analysis process, it should be reapplied to the data that has already been coded to ensure that all content was coded against the same criteria (White et al., 2006).

Train Coders and Assess Reliability and Validity

The final step to be performed in a content analysis—even though a content analysis is a fluid and iterative process, whereby you may return to a previous step, re-review data, recode, and refine your codebook—is to train additional coders or team members and evaluate quality assurance metrics, such as reliability and validity. Zolnoori et al. (2019) established specific criteria for coding and guidelines with examples of coded statements taken directly from the content that was used to maintain coding consistency and interrater reliability. Establishing coding guidelines is useful for training coders in the event that a team hires research assistants to help with data analysis.

Demonstrating scientific rigor and the quality of a content analysis is done by measuring several quality criteria, particularly reliability and validity (Cavanagh, 1997). Note that these metrics are specific to content analysis. Other criteria for which the rigor and quality of qualitative studies are evaluated are discussed in Chapter 5.

Reliability

In a content analysis, reliability is the extent to which more than one coder independently classifies content in the same way. Reliability is established by measuring the degree to which two raters agree on their coding, when this is done separately. These metrics are called interrater reliability, or interannotator agreement (IAA), and there are three primary formulas that are used to demonstrate a study adheres to this quality benchmark: percent agreement, Cohen's Kappa, and Krippendorff's Alpha. Reliability is often tied to reproducibility because it signals that data analysis can be reproduced in another study or the codebook can be reapplied to similar content. HIT studies often involve a multidisciplinary team. Working on a team enables multiple coders, which saves time and effort to perform data analysis. When dividing coding tasks among a team, the level of rigor can be questioned. McHugh (2012) states that, "Reliability of data collection is a component of overall confidence in a research study's accuracy," and is a quality of rigor for which research is evaluated for because it demonstrates that the phenomenon of interest is being evaluated and interpreted in the same way by multiple researchers. Variables subject to interrater errors can compromise the accuracy of qualitative research findings.

A reliability metric used to establish interrater reliability is used as evidence that individual raters are coding content according to the same categories. Often, interrater reliability is expressed as a percent agreement between two independent raters. To calculate percent agreement, simply sum the number of cases that were coded in the same way by the two raters and divide this number by the total number of cases that were coded. Khajouei et al. (2009) used percent agreement to support the reliability of the usability problems discovered by two independent evaluators during a cognitive walkthrough usability inspection of a computerized physician order entry (CPOE) system. The higher the percent agreement, the more reliable a study; however, the shortfall with using percent agreement is that it does not account for the fact that raters are expected to agree with each other some of the time by chance alone (Stemler, 2001).

Therefore, the more commonly used interrater reliability metric is Cohen's Kappa, which uses a scale from 0 to 1. When expressing interrater reliability using the Cohen's Kappa statistic, 1 means coding by individual raters has perfect agreement and 0 means there is no agreement except that by chance (Stemler, 2001). This metric is established by having two raters independently code a predefined number of content pieces or cases, then calculating Kappa using the following formula:

$$k = \frac{P_o - P_e}{1 - P_e} = 1 - \frac{1 - P_o}{1 - P_e},$$

P_o = the relative observed agreement among raters.

P_e = the hypothetical probability of chance agreement.

Krippendorff's Alpha (α) is a reliability coefficient that measures the agreement between two independent raters (Krippendorff, 2011). Krippendorff's Alpha can be a complex calculation, but fortunately there are SPSS packages that you can download to compute the coefficient for you, as well as many QDAS that will also calculate it for you. To calculate Krippendorff's Alpha, you first need to have a subsample of your data be coded independently by all the coders. The general formula is:

$$\alpha = 1 - \frac{D_o}{D_e}$$

D_o = the observed disagreement among values assigned to units of analysis.

D_e = the disagreement one would expect when the coding of units is attributable to chance rather than to the properties of these units.

Like Cohen's Kappa, the reliability using Krippendorff's Alpha is evaluated on a scale from 0 to 1, where

$\alpha = 1$ = perfect reliability

$\alpha = 0$ = absence of reliability

$\alpha < 0$ = disagreements are systematic and exceed what can be expected by chance (Krippendorff, 2004; 2011).

For more details on how to calculate Krippendorff's Alpha, see Krippendorff (2011), Oleinik et al. (2014), and Zapf et al. (2016), which offer steps to use in calculating the metric manually. If you need to argue for the reliability of your study findings, for instance, for the sake of a peer-reviewed publication, calculating the Kappa statistic or Krippendoff's coefficient may benefit your argument; however, when a study's purpose is to obtain useful insights that can be applied to design usability HIT or identify usability problems in existing HIT, it may not add value to your study.

Validity

Validity is the extent to which an instrument measures what it claims to measure. In a content analysis, construct validity is often established to show that a code or theme accurately represents the concept or aspect of the content that it is intended to represent. As discussed previously, construct validity is the extent to which a code or theme accurately represents or measures the concept being assessed (White et al., 2006). Creating a clear operational codebook and adhering to it will increase the validity of a study (Hsiu-Fang et al., 2005). Validity can also be established in a qualitative study in the form of triangulation. Triangulation lends credibility to the findings by incorporating multiple sources of data or investigators (Erlandson, 1993). Ensuring that you are collecting a large, heterogenous, representative sample, and describing the systematic process by which you collected your sample of content, will support the validity of your study.

Manifest versus Latent Content

One factor to consider when performing data analysis of qualitative data is whether you are going to code manifest and/or latent content. Manifest content is the exact, literal meaning of a word, passage of text, or verbal report transcription. One easy method of coding manifest content is to highlight or search for specific words or passages that exemplify that category or theme. When using QDAS, you can perform a word count to accelerate this process. A content analysis that only analyzes for the appearance of particular content is generally more quantitative in nature (Hsiu-Fang et al., 2005). Latent content is the underlying meaning behind the word, passage of text, or verbalization, body gestures, and facial expressions from subjects. "Latent content analysis refers to the process of interpretation" (Hsiu-Fang et al., 2005, p. 1283). When coding latent content of observational behavior, you do not necessarily code a "shrug" or "grimace" facial expression, but you would code the meaning behind the shrug or reason why the subject made the facial expression—for instance, perhaps you infer that they were confused or excited, or had a positive or negative reaction to specific content or HCI. When you abstract deeper layers of meaning beyond just the meaning of a word or gesture from a subject, such as silence, sighs, and laughter, you are analyzing latent content (Elo et al., 2014; Erlingsson et al., 2017).

CONTENT ANALYSIS IN A MIXED-METHODS STUDY

The purpose of this chapter was to demonstrate how content analysis can be used in a mixed-methods study of HIT to understanding existing health information, messages, or user interface content that is used for various purposes in HIT and to facilitate healthcare delivery through various health information systems. The coding techniques used during content analysis are applied when performing data analysis of qualitative data obtained from user research methods and usability testing, such as interviews and think-aloud usability tests. It is important that when coding, you focus on transforming the data into meaningful insight that helps you answer your research question or is useful from a practical standpoint, and can be used to drive refinements in HIT design that will improve usability. I encourage the blending of techniques, and reusing and expanding on HIT coding schemes that allow you to best represent the qualitative data you collect and describe the aspects of the phenomenon under investigation that your research questions define.

SUMMARY

This chapter described content analysis and its application in health research. Three different coding techniques were discussed and examples were provided to demonstrate how to perform each of the approaches to coding: deductive, inductive, and framework analysis. The most common quality assurance metrics used to evaluate content analysis studies were also introduced, including intercoder reliability and construct validity. The coding techniques discussed in this chapter will be referred to in subsequent chapters as they are applied when analyzing the empirical data obtained from many empirical research methods. Lastly, this chapter is intended to empower researchers and practitioners to build on previous research and mixed methods to be able to gain useful and valuable insight regarding the usability of HIT, such as to create new coding schemes to understand how patients perceive telemedicine when none exists.

7

Discovery UX Research Studies

INTRODUCTION

This chapter discusses the types of generative research that typically is conducted prior to the design of a HIT in order to define the problem that is being solved and deeply understand the target users for whom the HIT is being designed. Research that is generative is termed so because it collects data that offer insights about the target users, their needs, attitudes, and behaviors, and other contextual factors that are used to inform the design of a HIT that is actually going to be useful and usable for the target user population. Discovery research is qualitative in nature and there are no formalized, systematic ways of performing each method discussed in this chapter; therefore, a brief description of each method will be offered followed by references to existing research that has implemented that method. The primary methods discussed in this chapter are field studies, diary studies, focus groups, interviews, and surveys. Card sorting will also be described. There are many different ways of approaching the design of generative UX research methods, and it is recommended to always focus on your research questions and objectives, and design the study in ways that will best help you to answer your research questions and achieve your research objectives.

GENERATIVE VERSUS EVALUATIVE RESEARCH

Discovery research is generative and performed at the beginning of UCD or the full system design lifecycle because the aim is to understand the target user, the tasks they perform, and the goals they need to achieve when using a technology product or system, as well as to gain a rich account of the target user's context of use. Discovery research is often called exploratory because it seeks to deeply understand the target user, their pain points and problems, and their context,

DOI: 10.1201/9781003460886-7

which includes their environment and social, material, and organizational factors that may impact their interaction with technology—or a concept—as it may be that you are evaluating a conceptual technology (Yen et al., 2017). Evaluative methods aim to assess technology products (prototypes) to ensure usability based on the users' wants, needs, and desires.

FIELD STUDIES VERSUS LABORATORY STUDIES

The UX field is plagued with various terms and methods that mean the same thing or that are just slightly different. "Field studies" and "ethnography" are two terms that are often used to refer to the same method, and are used interchangeably. However, with regard to UX research, there are essentially only two types of studies: field studies or laboratory studies. Field studies are distinguished from laboratory studies by the way in which the researcher interacts with the user. In field studies, the researcher goes to the client or customer to observe users in their natural environment. Laboratory studies entail bringing the user (or participants) to a laboratory to test them or observe them interacting with a product in an environment that is not natural and probably unlike the context in which they would ever interact with the artifact being tested. Like all studies, there is a best use case for each to be implemented. Field studies are typically conducted at the beginning of the design of a new product or service, or during the UCD process. Laboratory studies are typically reserved for more formal usability testing or when specific UX research software or tools can only be used in a laboratory setting. Chapter 5 discusses the various study environments.

FIELD STUDIES

The field study, as mentioned previously, is a method that is highly variable and is often used interchangeably with ethnography. However, there are different variants of field studies and ethnography is just one of them. You can choose to embed yourself in the context and aspire to have a minimal impact on the individuals you are observing. Traditional ethnographic research entails the research embedding themselves on-site, in the context and environment of the user group they seek to understand. Besides knowing that the researcher is there, there is minimal, if no, interaction between the researcher and the people they are observing. The researcher is a silent observer. On the other hand, contextual inquiry is a type of field study where the researcher asks questions as they observe to gain clarity or more insight on certain observed behaviors.

Both approaches are beneficial and have limitations. With ethnography, you rely on the researcher's ability to make accurate interpretations of their observations and may not gain a rich, detailed understanding of the various social, organizational, cultural, and contextual factors that impact people's behavior. With contextual inquiry, you are able to gain a rich, detailed, and likely more accurate representation of the target user's context and interactions that occur in that context; however, because you interrupt the user to ask questions, you run the risk of disrupting a realistic workflow and people may be subject to the Hawthorne effect or other biases. The Hawthorne effect refers to people's tendency to change their behaviors when they know or feel they are being observed (McCambridge et al., 2014). Generally, as will be reminded and reinforced in every chapter, define your research questions or objectives, and select the best methods that will allow you to answer your research questions and achieve your research objectives. Field studies are flexible and there is no step-by-step process to conduct a field study; therefore, I will provide you a general overview of each approach and refer to existing research that entailed implementing each method.

Ethnography

The terms "ethnography" and "ethnographic research" originated in the social science discipline of anthropology. Ethnography \is the study of social interactions, behaviors, and perceptions that occur within groups, teams, organizations, and communities (Reeves et al., 2008). Ethnographic research yields rich, holistic insights into people's views and actions, as well as the nature (that is, sights and sounds) of the location they inhabit, through collecting detailed observations and interviews (Berg et al., 2004; Reeves et al., 2008). Ethnography is associated primarily with the work that anthropologists do, which comprises understanding and writing about communities or people who are under investigation. In UX research, ethnography is a method whereby the researcher goes into the "field" or target user's environment and is immersed in the context of the user to engage in purposeful observations (Ackerman et al., 2015). Ethnographic research is qualitative in nature and the data collected is in the form of field notes, audio, and/or video recordings.

Formal ethnography is structured within specific time periods and conducted by expert ethnographers or trained researchers to remain as objective as possible. "To minimize the effect of the observation on the behavior of the study participants, no data that could identify person, place, or time of day was collected nor was any demographic information or medication error rate informant recorded" (Rogers et al., 2005). Formal interviews may also be conducted with the people being investigated. Less-formal field studies include just hanging out and casual conversations. Reflexivity plays a large role in ethnography as the researcher(s) reflect on how their role in the participants' environment may have impacted or changed their words or behaviors as ethnography aims to present an accurate representation of the participants and their context, and understand the differences between what people say and what they do (Ackerman et al., 2015).

Despite ethnographic research being implemented in the health information technology space only in a limited way—mainly because it is time-intensive, requires UX practitioners to gain trust and approval to enter people's environment, and can be costly—it is increasingly being recognized as a valuable method to generate important insight into the complex social and material conditions that shape users' interactions with and adoption of HIT (Ackerman et al., 2015). Ethnography is recognized and promoted as a useful generative approach to implement in the UCD of HIT (Schumacher et al., 2010) as it is a method for engaging with users early in the design process and focusing on the tasks they need to accomplish (Gould et al., 1985). In fact, the U.S. Office of the National Coordinator for Health IT (ONC) lists ethnography, alongside contextual inquiry, as a method to get a rich picture of users, their context, and the environment, and includes ethnography in its design framework for EHR vendors to be able to meet usability certification requirements (Schumacher et al., 2010). Some of the research questions that can be answered by collecting data from field studies include:

- How is the HIT meant to fit within the organization?
- In what context will the HIT be accessed and used?
- Who will be the primary users and what are their goals for use?
- What is the intended users' experience with similar HIT?
- What are barriers to adoption of the HIT or for it to be successfully implemented? (Schumacher et al., 2010)

Ethnography is highly variable and flexible, yet all ethnographic studies of social and behavioral phenomena are conducted in naturalistic settings through observation; the researcher is embedded in the social world of the users they aim to study, and thus uniquely observes behaviors as they occur in situ (Morgan-Trimmer & Wood, 2016). The number of people being observed can vary depending on the artifact and phenomenon under investigation and the location of the field study. There can be as few as one or two people being observed, or several (40 to 100) users can be observed in settings where many people congregate, such as in the setting of an emergency department (ED) (Fabricius et al., 2021) or Intensive Care Unit (ICU) (Leslie et al., 2017). Observation periods can be as little as a few hours, or they can be days, months, or years (Fabricius et al., 2021; Leslie et al., 2017; Rogers et al., 2005). Often, the observation period is followed by interviews with key participants. Between 10 and 12 participants per user group (patients, nurses, physicians, etc.) should be recruited to participate in interviews conducted to gain a clearer understanding of the phenomena under investigation (Fabricius et al., 2021; Leslie et al., 2017). Findings from ethnographic research are often triangulated with findings from other methods or used to inform the execution of other methods, such as in the development of an interview guide for conducting interviews. A few ethnographic studies in the healthcare space are described next.

Leslie et al. (2017) performed a mixed-methods comparative study of three ICUs to examine the aggregate of work using HIT and its influence on shaping clinical relationships. A total of 446 hours of non-participant observations were conducted in three different ICUs over the course of a one-year observational period (Leslie et al., 2017). "Fly on the wall" observational data was collected in the form of field notes (Leslie et al., 2017). Informal interviews with the staff and patients occurred during natural breaks in the ICU workflow so as not to disrupt the natural activities and behaviors of the people who were being observed (Leslie et al., 2017). The ethnographic research was followed by job-shadowing 47 participants, consisting of 32 nurses and 15 junior doctors who worked in the ICU, to log their HIT usage by minute (Leslie et al., 2017).

Similarly, because Pope et al. (2013) sought to perform a comparative study of how the use of a CDSS did or did not become a part of routine practice in three different healthcare settings, ethnography was their method of choice as it allowed them to explore the context and behaviors of the users in their nature environment. "This method was chosen to capture the complexities of social interaction in a naturalistic rather than experimental way" (Pope et al., 2013). Non-participant observation in three different healthcare facilities was conducted over a 20-month period, at different times of the day. Although the focus of the observational research was on the call-handlers using the CDSS, Pope et al. (2013) were able to observe several other clinical staff, such as clinical supervisors and ambulance dispatchers, who may or may not have interacted with the CDSS, in their natural context, thus obtaining a rich, detailed data set in the form of detailed notes. The qualitative data captured included details of the activities of the users of the CDSS, times of the day, and transcribed verbatim or near-verbatim statements from the people they observed (Pope et al., 2013). In addition to the field notes, Pope et al. (2013) conducted informal and semi-structured interviews with other stakeholders (policy-makers and managers, among others). The interview guide was developed based on what was learned during the non-participant observational research (Pope et al., 2013). Pope et al.'s (2013) research team consisted of individuals from an array of social science backgrounds using the theoretical lens of normalization process theory to examine and uncover the ways in which the CDSS became embedded in the everyday work practices of various clinical staff.

Rizvi et al. (2017) performed a mixed-methods study including ethnographic research because the "approach to data collection provides rich, realistic, and holistic view of user behavior in task completion and could aid in gathering additional detailed information, which users sometimes fail to communicate during more controlled (e.g., laboratory based) methodological approaches" (Rizvi et al., 2017, p. 1096). To understand how the clinical notes feature of two EHR systems impacted usability, Rizvi et al., (2017) conducted ethnographic research by immersing themselves in the physicians' environment and observing their daily routine activities and interactions with the EHRs. To ensure a representative sample of observational data could be obtained, each physician was observed on various days of the week and weekend, and in various sections of the clinic, for four to five days in total (Rizvi et al., 2017). About two to two and a half hours of observation time was logged during the daytime hours, totaling over 110 hours spent in observation (Rizvi et al., 2017). To obtain additional subjective data, a post-observation questionnaire was deployed to participants (Rizvi et al., 2017). The qualitative data were collected using the Timestamped Field Notes application on a tablet (Rizvi et al., 2017).

Fabricius et al. (2021) performed an ethnographic study seeking to explore the determinants of patient involvement in decisions about their medication before implementing shared decision-making. In the context of two medical EDs, 48 various health professionals were observed for 58 days (Fabricius et al., 2021). Each participant was observed for an average of three hours per day during the observation period (Fabricius et al., 2021). A total of 144 hours of observational data, including verbal and nonverbal reactions, was collected in the form of detailed textual material (Fabricius et al., 2021). Using findings from the ethnographic research, Fabricius et al. (2021) developed an interview guide to conduct interviews with 10 healthcare professionals who participated in the ethnographic study and 10 who had not participated to validify their interpretations of the field observations.

Most ethnographic data undergo thematic data analysis using an inductive approach to identify key themes and issues that emerge from the data, generating explanations for their empirical work (Reeves et al., 2008). As such, ethnographers practice reflectivity—constant elucidation of the acts involved in the inquiry process (Mortari, 2015)—and reflexivity—understanding of the relationship a researcher shares with the world they are investigating (Reeves et al., 2008)—to ensure methodological rigor and that an accurate interpretation has been made of the context and interactions, attitudes, behaviors, and beliefs of the people being observed.

Contextual Inquiry

A sister to ethnography is contextual inquiry, which allows the researcher to obtain more details about specific observations, such as behaviors of the users or attitudes regarding certain interactions, because it entails the researcher inquiring about certain contextual aspects with the users and participating in the discovery process by asking questions. Contextual inquiry is a field of study that involves participant observation—a mode for gaining insight into the meaning permeating people's daily lives and activities by constant self-reflective participation and extensive observation (Gans, 1999).

Contextual inquiry can be performed in a formal, structured format, in a semi-structured format, or in a flexible format where questions are asked only when needed. Beyer and Holtzblatt (1998, p. 22) assert that "the first problem for design is to understand the customers: their needs, their desires, their approach to the work." Contextual inquiry is a field interviewing method that addresses this problem by applying open-ended qualitative interview techniques that make explicit unarticulated knowledge about a target user's work and the structure of work practice, including low-level details that are often invisible (Beyer et al., 1998). Both ethnography and contextual inquiry aim to understand target users in context, which is more representative of their work, context, and how they might interact with technology. Yet the main distinction between traditional ethnography and contextual inquiry is the difference between the researcher acting like a "fly on the wall," and not participating in the observation activity or interacting with the participants as they observe them, and acting as an apprentice as they perform a task (Beyer et al., 1998).

Contextual techniques are designed to gather data from customers in the field, where people are working or living. Contextual inquiry is a field data-gathering technique that studies a few carefully selected individuals in depth to arrive at a fuller understand of the work practice across all customers. Through inquiry and interpretation, it reveal commonalities across a system's customer base.

(Beyer et al., 1998)

The following principles guide the implementation of contextual inquiry in practice:

- *Context.* This principle asserts that it is important to go to the setting of the users you want to observe so you can gather ongoing experiential, concrete data rather than summary, often abstract data.
- *Partnership.* Partnership refers to the way in which you will collaborate with the user to understand their work. The power tilts toward the interviewer in traditional interviewing, but when you are partnered with your participant, you interact and exchange rich knowledge about their behaviors and attitudes.
- *Interpretation.* Interpretation is key all qualitative data collection and analysis. Interpretation is the chain of reasoning that turns observational data into a meaningful insight.
- *Focus.* Focus defines the point of view an interviewer takes while studying a context and phenomena. Focus allows the interviewer to guide the conversation with the user to topics that are going to be useful (Beyer et al., 1998).

Because contextual inquiry has you collaborate with the user in an intimate way, it is treated much like interviews and about 10 to 12 participants will be recruited to participate in a contextual inquiry session. Additionally, data saturation is often reached during the data analysis of contextual inquiry and interview data (Hendriks et al., 2022). The duration of a contextual inquiry session is longer than an interview might be, such as over the course of a participant's workday or a few hours a day for several days, weeks, months, or years depending on the phenomena under investigation. A typical contextual inquiry, like an interview, has the researcher begin with an introduction and some general questions about the participant's situation and then proceed to the observation and discussion of the task under investigation (Hendriks et al., 2022).

Contextual inquiry was performed by Jalil et al. (2019) to investigate how to uncover a patient's user experience as it related to their use of telehealth,

eHealth, and mHealth in a clinical trial. Nine patients who had type 2 diabetes mellitus (T2D) were recruited to participate in the in situ study that occurred at their regularly scheduled time to use a tablet computer that sent their medical data (blood glucose reading, blood pressure) to the clinical trial team (Jalil et al., 2019). In addition, five family members provided occasional feedback (Jalil et al., 2019). Immediately following the contextual inquiry, a semi-structured interview was conducted with each participant, and a follow-up survey was sent to each participant eight months after the initial study to see whether there were any changes with the patients' use of the device (Jalil et al., 2019). The contextual inquiry and interviews were audio-recorded, and the recordings were transcribed (Jalil et al., 2019). Contextual inquiry data also included field notes (Jalil et al., 2019). Although Jalil et al. (2019) note that they had a small sample size and that a larger sample of T2D participants would need to participate in future work in order to generalize the findings across this population, they also advocated for the value of contextual inquiry and in situ studies as they are able to capture the patient's perspective and paint a better picture of the HCI that occurs between patients and HIT.

Likewise, Hendriks et al. (2022) performed contextual inquiry as a part of a mixed-methods study with 10 adults who sought to quit smoking through the use of an app. The study's aim was to better understand people's experience and needs as they search for mobile apps for smoking cessation (Hendriks et al., 2022). The contextual inquiry sessions took place at various locations in order to be a natural setting for participants, including in their homes and workplaces (Hendriks et al., 2022). Audio and screen recordings were captured during the contextual inquiry and field notes were also taken (Hendriks et al., 2022). Each contextual inquiry session was for a different duration, with the shortest being 50 minutes and the longest being over two hours (Hendriks et al., 2022). Two weeks after the contextual inquiry, participants were interviewed in a semi-structured format (Hendriks et al., 2022). An interview guide was used to conduct the interviews, which lasted from 10 to 34 minutes (Hendriks et al., 2022). The qualitative data collected included audio and screen recordings, and thematic analysis was used to analyze this raw data (Hendriks et al., 2022). Additional quantitative data were collected, such as the number of apps that participants looked at (Hendriks et al., 2022). In adherence to the apprenticeship principle of contextual inquiry, "After the participants made their final choice for an app, we jointly created a summary of the entire search process. Doing this together with the participant served as a means of checking our interpretations" (Hendriks et al., 2022).

DIARY STUDIES

Diary studies are likely one of the least frequently employed methods in healthcare UX research. A diary study is a longitudinal research method that aims to capture situated practices in users' natural environment by having them record entries about their everyday lives about the phenomena under investigation (Jarrahi et al., 2021; Wildemuth, 2017). As the name implies, diary studies traditionally involved participants keeping a written track record of activities, events, and their behaviors, attitudes, and sentiment at different times during the diary study (Wildemuth, 2017). However, given the digital resources and tools available today, diary studies have emerged as a very versatile method for capturing both qualitative and quantitative measurements of a UX. That said, generally diary studies would be considered more a qualitative research method because they aim to capture the lived, subjective experience of people as they move through the events of their daily lives (Bolger et al., 2003). Also known as "ecological momentary assessment," diary studies ask subjects to report on their environment, such as their location and the presence of others; their perceptions of their environment, such as the stressfulness of a situation; and internal states or moods, such as fear, excitement, or angst, among other aspects that a researcher desires to understand about a UX (Ciere et al., 2015; Shiffman et al., 2008).

Because diary studies are longitudinal—that is, they are completed over the course of a long time period, and because they require subjects to maintain an intensive measurement schedule, they can be difficult to implement in the study of HIT or a healthcare context. However, they have many strengths that make them a viable method to use if one seeks to understand a UX in a real-world context. Diary studies offer four primary affordances:

- *In situity:* they maximize ecological validity because they take place in subjects' natural environment.
- *Context specificity:* they allow for the discovery of microprocesses that influence behavior in real-world contexts.
- *Longitudinally:* they take place over time and can expose changes that short duration studies might not.
- *Minimize recall bias:* they allow for subjects to reflect and report on their experience as it unfolds, in real-time (Bolger et al., 2003; Jarrahi et al., 2021).

Qualitative research sample sizes vary and largely depend on the nature and scope of the study, as well as the resources available to perform the study, such as funding and accessibility of representative users. Synthesizing a variety of resources suggests that to obtain rich, detailed data, a small sample size of six to 12 subjects is sufficient. For a more exploratory-focused study, where the aim is to understand the major and breadth of themes related to a UX, a larger sample size of 30 to 60 participants would be considered rigorous (Mason, 2010; Morse, 1994, 2000; Subedi, 2021). The duration of diary studies depends on the phenomena being investigated.

> According to the principle of longitudinality, the time frame for the study should be based on the expected amount of time needed for the phenomenon under study to occur. As such, selecting the time frame is a careful balance between minimizing effort for participants and maximizing results.
>
> (Jarrahi et al., 2021)

For instance, if a research objective is to evaluate an individual's change of behavior over time, it would be necessary to ask participants to retrospect over several weeks and months and provide summary accounts of their psychological states, behaviors, and experiences (Bolger et al., 2003), whereas if the focus of the study was to understand individuals' use of their mobile devices within their workday, then participants might only be required to submit diary entries twice a day over the course of seven days (Jarrahi et al., 2021).

Daniëls et al. (2021) report on the factors that influence the use of diary studies in the healthcare space in a scoping review. The factors were categorized into three main themes: intervention (data collection instrument, look and feel, functionalities, and performance), user characteristics (sociodemographic information, attitudes, skills and knowledge, and motivation), and process (training and instructions). Considering the ability of diary studies to capture the lived experience of individuals, including their mood and behaviors, they are highly applicable in the healthcare space and to capture individuals' perceptions when using HIT, and are being leveraged more in the industry because of tools such as Indeemo (Twohig, 2022) and dscout (dscout, 2023).

Both Bradway et al. (2020) and Blödt et al. (2014) conducted a diary study for one part of a mixed-methods study of patients use of mHealth apps to facilitate shared-decision making with their healthcare provider (Bradway et al., 2020) and self-treat chronic low back and neck pain through relaxation. Both studies utilized an app as the data collection instrument and intervention being investigated. Bradway et al. (2020) leveraged a pre-existing, validated Diabetes Diary mobile phone app that allows patients to register their self-gathered health measurements (blood glucose and physical activity), review previously registered data, and share and view their personal health information (PHI) with their healthcare provider. In Blödt et al.'s (2014) study, an app was developed to provide the audio relaxation content for patients and collect the data required to achieve their research objective, which was to evaluate whether an additional mHealth-delivered intervention was more effective in the reduction of chronic lower back pain or neck pain than traditional care alone.

Bradway et al.'s (2020) diary study recruited 23 participants—13 general practitioners (GPs), two nurses, and eight patients—from two different hospitals. Participants were encouraged to use the Diabetes Diary app during the six-month study time period and were also tasked with completing a post-consultation questionnaire each time they visited their GP and participate in a post-study focus group in order to measure their self-management habits and perceived health status and challenges that they may have with the self-management of diabetes parameters (Bradway et al, 2020).

Similarly, Blödt et al.'s (2014) study leveraged a mobile app to both present the intervention and collect the diary self-reports reflections from patients as they used the mobile app intervention. To evaluate whether the intervention had an effect size of 0.4, Blödt et al. (2014) calculated that at least 100 participants were required for each treatment group (mHealth intervention and no intervention). Therefore, 110 participants per treatment group were recruited to compensate for dropouts (Blödt et al., 2014). The study was completed over a six-month time period (Blödt et al., 2014). Participants were instructed to use the mobile intervention for 15 minutes per day for at least five days in a week (Blödt et al., 2014). Baseline data were collected in the traditional format, on paper, and follow-up data were collected daily, weekly, and after three and six months using the digital diary built into the mobile app (Blödt et al., 2014).

FOCUS GROUPS

Focus groups (or group interviews) are a sociological method that relies on group dynamics to facilitate the construction of knowledge by gathering in-depth, subjective information from a small group of individuals (Billson, 1989). The concept of group dynamics refers to the shared social context's ability to encourage group members to become involved and voice their views and opinions. Focus groups, interviews, and surveys are the top-most leveraged qualitative method for soliciting information about users' impressions and perspectives on various topics or their use of HIT, for gathering information about users' needs, and for eliciting ideas for the improvement of HIT or healthcare delivery (Yen et al., 2012). The goal of focus groups is to elicit and garner a range of opinions regarding a certain object of investigation, which is beneficial in the discovery stages of the full system design lifecycle.

To facilitate a focus group, at least one moderator is needed. Often the PI is the moderator. Focus groups are a data gathering technique that relies on the systematic questioning of several individuals simultaneously in a formal or informal setting (Fontana & Frey, 2000). Like interviews, focus groups can be structured, semi-structured, or unstructured (where the discussion is more free-flowing). A moderator's guide can be developed to support the facilitation of the focus groups and list questions that should be addressed. Focus groups are typically audio-recorded to capture the participants' verbal reports. Between six and 10 participants should be recruited to participate in focus groups (Billson, 1989; Krueger & Casey, 2009).

Mixed-methods studies often include a focus group session at the beginning (as exploratory research) or end (as confirmatory research) of a study because they afford an easy way to gather additional subjective user feedback that can be used to triangulate the findings from other methods or corroborate other findings.

There are many examples of mixed-methods studies in the healthcare space that leverage focus groups (Doran et al., 2007; Eysenbach et al., 2002; Schmidt-Kraepelin et al., 2014; Whitehead et al., 2007; Zulman et al., 2015). A few examples will be discussed next. Doran et al. (2007) conducted 12 focus group sessions that included between two and nine nurse participants to understand how nurses collect and utilize information to make decisions at the point of patient care. Schmidt-Kraepelin et al. (2014) conducted four focus groups targeting eight participants and utilized a structured format facilitated by a moderator guide (the authors referred to the topic guide and questioning route (Krueger, 1998) to elicit users' perspective of the usability of ePill, a patient-centered HIT. Whitehead et al. (2007) conducted focus groups with hospital staff and then surveyed hospital in-patients to corroborate the data collected from the focus group sessions in a mixed-methods study aiming to identify the key factors that influence patients' perceptions of cleanliness in a hospital setting. Two focus groups were conducted, each consisting of six to eight participants (Whitehead et al., 2007).

INTERVIEWS

A plethora of mixed-methods studies in the healthcare space leverage interviews as one of the primary qualitative methods to explore and understand the UX

(Khairat et al., 2019; Peters & Halcomb, 2015; Yen et al., 2012). Yen et al. (2012) found that interviews were used in all stages of the full system design lifecycle to explore and measure system specifications, HCIs, and user perceptions, as well as utilization and patient outcomes. Interviews entail talking to representative/target users about their experience by asking them a series of open-ended questions that surround a topic or subject matter. Interviews are often the first method used in user-centered frameworks such as UCD and design thinking because they involve users immediately, at the start of the full system design lifecycle, which is recommended by design experts (Dumas et al., 1999; Gould et al., 1985). However, interviews are also employed throughout and in the latter stages of the full system design lifecycle because they capture users' perceptions after using a HIT and insights from users can also support findings from other methods used, such as usability tests or surveys.

Structured interviews means that the same questions are asked to participants in the same order, with no other probing from the interviewer to obtain further details. Structured interviews may qualify as more rigorous because they are conducted in a more systematic way, but semi-structured interviews are often a better way of collecting rich data and gaining an in-depth understanding of the UX. Semi-structured interviews mean that some predefined questions or topics to be addressed have been established, but the interviewer probes further as the participant responds (Peters et al., 2015), asking them to clarify, elaborate, or provide more details to gain richer data.

Both structured and semi-structured interviews are based on an interview guide, developed by the researcher(s), which is a schematic presentation of the questions, topics, or needs to be explored by the interviewer (Dicicco-Bloom & Crabtree, 2006). An interview guide, like other research protocols, should start with an introduction to the research and an explanation of the risks and benefits to the participants. Following an informed consent section, the interview guide lists the questions or topics that will be addressed in the interview.

The qualitative data collected during interviews are in the form of audio- and sometimes video-recordings, however, the data analyzed comes only from the verbal reports from participants. Notes taken by the researcher or a silent interlocutor may aid in data analysis. Interviews are transcribed verbatim or near verbatim and undergo a thematic analysis to uncover themes or key factors relating to the phenomenon being investigated, which generate meaningful findings.

For generative/discovery research, 10 to 12 participants should be recruited to be interviewed (Fox, 2016; Vasileiou et al., 2018; Virzi, 1992), which is the sample size where data saturation seems to be achieved. If the aim of the research is to be able to make generalizations or comparisons across variables, then a larger sample of 20 to 30 participants is recommended. Often user personas and user journey maps are developed in the early discovery stages of UCD or in the development of a new product or service, and it is estimated that at least five interviewees are needed per user group for which a persona is developed (Rosala, 2021)—for example, if you were examining the user experience of clinicians' use of telemedicine, as Indria et al. (2020) did in their study. Clinicians are a broad user population that consists of several different user groups, which could be distinguished on the basis of specialty medicine practiced, years in practice, practice location, patient population, and more. For each specific target user group for which you were going to develop a user persona, you would need to recruit at least five clinicians who were representative of that user group to participate in an interview. Considering that clinicians are one of the primary users of telemedicine and their perspective has a great impact on the implementation and widespread adoption of telemedicine, Indria et al. (2020) sought to understand clinicians' perspective of telemedicine using mixed-methods consisting of a survey and semi-structured interviews.

A purposive sampling technique was used to recruit general practitioners, nurses, and midwives in Makassar City and surrounding areas to complete the survey, which was developed to assess clinicians' overall perception of using telemedicine (Indria et al., 2020). Three open-ended questions solicited clinicians' free-response feedback on what aspects of telemedicine they liked and disliked, and what future improvements could be made (Indria et al., 2020). One hundred participants completed the questionnaire; of these, 15 were selected and asked to participate in in-depth interviews, which were conducted to gain more in-depth, rich data and triangulate with the findings from the questionnaire (Indria et al., 2020). Semi-structured interviews were conducted in a one-on-one, face-to-face format using seven questions to guide the interviewees to describe their experience using telemedicine and explain their perception of the benefits of and barriers to using telemedicine (Indria et al., 2020). In-depth interviews were conducted with 10 general practitioners and five nurses (Indria et al., 2020). The interview subjects were chosen because of their seniority and better knowledge of the telemedicine system (Indria et al., 2020). The qualitative data from the survey and interviews underwent thematic analysis to identify important themes surrounding clinicians' experience of telemedicine (Indria et al., 2020).

Interviewing primary target users or representative users is often done at the beginning and end of the full system design lifecycle or paired with other methods in mixed-methods studies. Much scientific literature in the healthcare and health informatics space involves interviews (Choi et al., 2014;

Eysenbach et al., 2002; Johnson et al., 2005; Martínez-Alcalá et al., 2013). In mixed-methods research, the interview method is either applied prior to or subsequently to other methods, including focus groups, usability tests, health assessments, and surveys, among others, because these methods are well suited to exploring a phenomenon and gaining an in-depth understanding of end-users' experiences, opinions, expectations, needs, pain points, and individual and subjective usability factors either before (Schaaf et al., 2020) or after (Sloan et al., 2022) they use a HIT in a real-world setting.

SURVEYS

The next method discussed, survey methodology, is often employed at the beginning of the full system design lifecycle to obtain feedback from a large population of representative users because it can be a quick, easy, and cost-effective method of soliciting user-feedback from a large sample size. In addition, surveys are often sent to target users following their participation in a study to understand the efficacy of a treatment or program, usability of a HIT, and to collect user insights regarding UX. Thus, like interviews, surveys are a common method of data collection in healthcare UX research and are often combined with other data collection methods in mixed-methods research (Whitten et al., 2007). There is a misconception that surveys are only quantitative in nature. While surveys can be developed to only include questions that collect quantitative data, such as multiple choice, ranking, yes or no, or Likert scales, surveys using free-response, open-ended questions collect qualitative data, and these types of surveys can be a valuable method to employ in the discovery stage of UX research.

Surveys afford researchers the flexibility to make quick changes to the content and can be deployed via many different mediums using various survey platforms, such as Qualtrics, SurveyMonkey, and Google Forms. Additionally, data can also be collected using a hard copy, pen-and-paper method and completed by participants in person.

The data collected from surveys can be qualitative, quantitative, or both. Because surveys are easy to develop and deploy, are generally low in cost, and are able to be quickly changed, they afford researchers an extremely flexible method of obtaining UX insights. Langbecker et al. (2017) summarize the strengths of survey methodology:

- Survey questions can be developed in a way that will capture individuals' experiences, perceptions, and attitudes.
- Participants' anonymity and confidently can be maintained and protected, so the participants' views and experiences can be independently analyzed and compared without jeopardizing relationships or revealing personally identifiable information and personal health information (PHI).
- Pre-existing scales can be used across studies, enabling the comparison and replication of results.
- The ability to collect data from large sample sizes at a low cost produces generalizable results and a holistic understanding of the target user population.
- The validity and reliability of survey instruments can be assessed through rigorous, transparent and well-accepted validation methods, which provides evidence that the survey instruments accurately measure the intended constructs they are to measure.

This chapter discusses surveys that are implemented at the beginning of an exploratory study and how to develop a novel survey. Existing, standardized, and validated post-study surveys will be discussed in Chapter 10.

To develop a survey, you must have established your research questions and objectives so you can develop survey questions that are able to capture the information you want participants to provide. Once identifying the constructs you want to measure or the key information you want to gather, you should develop questions that will be understood easily by participants and responded to in a way that best captures the data you want to collect.

There are various responses you can select to have participants provide you (yes/no; true/false; multiple choice; drop-down options; check-boxes; ranking; free response; Likert scales; and more) and the complexity with which you format the survey depends on the tool you are using. For instance, you can randomize the presentation of questions presented to respondents, you can make require responses to some questions and make others optional, and/or you can format the survey to have each question presented to respondents at a time or all questions presented at once.

SurveyMonkey allows you to download an entire survey as a PDF to be printed and completed using a pen-and-paper format. Qualtrics has implemented logic where you can have some questions appear and be presented to participants only after they have selected a specific response to a previous question that would prompt the follow-up question. For example, if you are evaluating a smoking cessation digital health intervention and want to first understand if your respondents smoke, you might ask a "Yes/No" question: "Do you smoke tobacco?" If "Yes" is selected, the next free response or multiple choice question that appears can be "How many cigarettes do you smoke per day?" If "No" is selected, the participant would move on to the next group of questions.

After a summary of research and an informed consent section (see Figure 7.1 for an example), surveys typically begin by asking participants questions that will capture demographic information and other background, individual information that may be relevant to the phenomena under investigation.

Common demographic and individual information that healthcare-specific surveys may ask for include gender, age, disease, diagnosis date, title, specialty healthcare practice, years in practice, knowledge of a particular intervention or tool, and more. It is recommended to pilot survey questions with a group of representative users prior to the deploying the survey to ensure construct validity (Katusiime et al., 2016).

In exploratory studies and for generalizable results, surveys should aim for about 100 respondents or more; however, this really depends on your target population of representative users. If your target user population is small, then your sample size might also be smaller. UX experts suggest that only 40 to 50 participants may be enough to obtain the insights you want to gain (Budiu et al., 2021; Campbell et al., 2021; Sauro, 2015; Sauro & Lewis, 2016; 2023). Generally, the more responses you can collect, the more rigorous your study is considered to be, but you may find that data saturation is achieved after analyzing a certain number of participants. If your target population is multifaceted and large, it is recommended to recruit or send out your survey to as many

Teledoc Website Usability Survey

Teledoc Website Usability Survey

The purpose of this survey is to find out how easy it is to use and understand the information on the Teledoc website. You will first be asked basic demographic data and then asked to go to www.teledoc.com, which is the Teledoc website. You will be asked a series of questions that has you look for information on the website and describe your experience with "yes" or "no" and free text responses to the questions.

Your responses are confidential and your privacy will be maintained. No personal identification information can be ascertained. You are free to withdraw at any time, and your data will not be retained.

Thank you for your participation.

FIGURE 7.1
Teledoc Website Usability Survey (Campbell, 2020b; Campbell et al., 2021) summary of research and informed consent section. Novel survey developed in SurveyMonkey by Campbell (2020b).

potential end-users in your target population as possible, because being able to collect 100 responses depends on the response rate (Sauro et al., 2016).

Other considerations when determining sample size are the confidence level and effect size. Effect size is the strength of the relationship between the independent variable and the dependent variable (Vaske et al., 2002). Confidence levels refer to the level of confidence you are willing to accept that the outcome observed is a result of the variable you are evaluating—or the percentage of time you are willing to accept that your hypothesis will be incorrect (Budiu, 2021; Vaske et al., 2002). Sauro and Lewis offer many calculators for researchers to calculate confidence intervals and sample sizes on their *MeasuringU* website (https://measuringu.com/calc).

Lee et al.'s (2015) study is a good example of research that leveraged survey methodology to understand the navigation needs of a large, multifaceted population of consumers who have chronic health conditions when seeking health information online. Using the insights gained from a previous qualitative study (Lee et al., 2014), Lee et al. (2015) developed questions that were able to collect the type of UX insights pertaining to their navigational needs that they wanted to capture, and tested them for construct validity with a pilot group of users. Additionally, the final survey included validated, standardized instruments for measuring eHealth literacy—the eHealth Literacy Scale (eHEALS)—and patient activation—PAM-13—to further explore how health literacy and patients' level of their ability to manage their own health and wellbeing impacted their navigational needs when seeking online health information (Lee et al., 2015).

In order to obtain our target of 400 submitted questionnaires, a total of 1104 individuals were invited by ResearchNow from their diverse participant pool (Lee et al., 2015). Of these 1104 individuals, 1027 agreed to participate (93.03 percent consent) (Lee et al., 2015). Of the 1027 individuals, 514 individuals (50.05 percent) met our eligibility criteria, and 400 (77.82 percent) completed the questionnaire (Lee et al., 2015).

From the survey results, Lee et al. (2015) were able to determine that approximately half of the population of consumers living with chronic health conditions have poor navigational skills when seeking health information online and could benefit from support in finding quality health information online.

Similarly, Sloan et al. (2022) unitized survey methodology combined with in-depth interviews to understand patients' and physicians' acceptance and perceptions of safety of telemedicine for rheumatology following the COVID-19 pandemic, which necessitated a rapid global transition to use telemedicine. Sloan et al. (2022) recruited a large sample size of patients who reported to be diagnosed with a rheumatological condition through multiple disease support groups. A variety of healthcare professionals involved in the care of rheumatology patients, including consultants, registrars, specialist nurses and GPs, were invited to participate in the survey disseminated through various rheumatology networks, such as the British Society for Rheumatology (Sloan et al., 2022). Sloan et al. (2022) were able to recruit 1340 patient participants and 111 clinician participants. They were able draw comparisons between patients and clinicians' experiences of telemedicine from the results of the survey.

In addition to Lee et al. (2015)'s study, other scientific literature that discuss the development of novel survey instruments includes Campbell et al. (2021) and Langbecker et al. (2017).

SUMMARY

This chapter discussed common generative research methods, including field studies, diary studies, group/individual interviews, and surveys. Generative research is conducted at the start of UCD as it collects insights about the target user and their context, which is used to inform the design of a HIT that is going to be successful when implemented. Generative research may also be referred to as exploratory or discovery research as the aim is to understand a phenomenon or problem in depth so HIT solutions can be designed to be useable and effective. The type of data collected during discovery research is most often qualitative and analyzed using various content analysis techniques discussed in Chapter 6. Post-study quantitative, standardized surveys and UX scales will be discussed in Chapter 10.

8

Usability Inspection Methods

INTRODUCTION

This chapter describes more traditional formative usability testing methods, such as those conducted with experts only and those conducted with end-users who act as subjects in a usability test. The three common formative usability inspections covered in this chapter are heuristic evaluations, cognitive walkthroughs, and think-aloud usability tests. A protocol is provided for each method, including how to approach study design and how many experts or subjects are recommended for each method. This chapter will end with a list of other cognitive approaches to evaluating the usability of HIT.

USABILITY INSPECTION METHODS

Usability inspection methods (UIMs) are any technique or method by which a system or interface is evaluated for the purpose of identifying usability problems or issues that affect end-users (Gray & Salzman, 1998; Nielsen & Landauer, 1993). The ultimate goal of performing usability inspections is to identify areas where the usability of a system or application can be improved. As discussed in Chapter 7, usability evaluations and user testing are evaluative methods, in contrast to the generative methods performed at the beginning of the full system design lifecycle. Evaluative research aims to test an existing solution to the problem defined from the findings produced by generative research.

Considering that human interaction with HIT has a profound impact on users' cognitive processes, there are a number of cognitive approaches to assessing HIT that borrow from cognitive psychology, computer science, and systems engineering (Kushniruk et al., 2004). The objective of evaluating usability in the formative stages of the full system design lifecycle is to understand the

DOI: 10.1201/9781003460886-8

"why" and "what" of the things people do when interacting with a technology product. To understand the how and why of humans' interaction with technology, usability experts and practitioners employ a variety of methods that "borrow from an interdisciplinary perspective and draw from a number of areas including cognitive psychology, computer science, systems engineering, and the field of usability engineering" (Kushniruk et al., 2004). Conventional summative and outcome-based usability evaluations lack the ability to identify the potential negative implications of HIT on humans' cognitive processes and are outside the scope of the iterative design process where usability problems can be fixed before the final product is released.

There are two types of usability inspection methods: exert-based and user-based. Expert-based involve a subject matter expert (SME) or usability expert, and user-based involve a representative user. User-based usability inspection methods are often called user testing or empirical research, and can be conducted in many ways depending on the study context and objective. The goals standard of usability testing method, the think-aloud protocol, is the only user-based usability testing method discussed in this chapter. Other methods used to evaluate usability are discussed at the end of this chapter and in subsequent chapters.

HEURISTIC EVALUATION

A heuristic evaluation is an expert-based usability inspection of a system or user interface that involves having usability experts review an interface against a set of established usability guidelines or principles, called "heuristics." Heuristic evaluations are often called formal expert reviews because they involve usability experts reviewing an application or user interface by focusing on a set of heuristics or design principles. Formal expert reviews are more systematic, whereas informal expert reviews entail usability experts simply evaluating a user interface (UI) holistically and identifying features, functions, or aspects of the UI that present potential usability problems based on their own expertise and knowledge.

Several usability heuristics have been developed to evaluate various user interfaces. The most well-known and most-used are Nielsen's 10 usability heuristics (Nielsen et al., 1990; Nielsen, 1994b). Other practitioners have developed additional or different usability principles for specific user interfaces or genres, such as Weinschenk and Barker's (2000) 20 usability principles for speech interfaces; the eight golden rules of interface design (Shneiderman, 1987); Tognazzini's (2014) first principles of interaction design; Gerhardt-Powals's (1996) 10 cognitive-design principles; 25 heuristics for evaluating mHealth apps developed by Khowaja and Al-Thani (2020); and 12 usability heuristics for evaluating touchscreen mobile devices (Weinsc Inostroza et al., 2012). Additionally, other scholars have developed usability heuristics specifically to be applied to HIT. Carvalho et al. (2009) identified 12 usability heuristics that were critical for patient safety when evaluating HISs, such as computerized physician order entry (CPOE) and decision support systems. Zhang et al. (2003) merged Nielsen's (1994b) 10 heuristics with Shneiderman's (1987) eight and added a few based on their own expertise to create a list of 14 usability heuristics to be applied in usability evaluations of medical devices. Monkman and Kushniruk (2013a) developed 29 evidence-based usability heuristics for evaluating the usability of consumer mHealth applications for populations with limited health literacy. A list of 14 evidence-based usability heuristics has been developed to be applied to telemedicine UIs (Campbell, 2023), such as consumer-facing telemedicine websites and their mobile UIs.

Heuristics are presented as a list of criteria and descriptions that usability experts can use to guide their evaluation. Krawiec and Dudycz (2020) compared several different usability heuristics and note that they often overlap or differ merely in terminology.

In general, during formal heuristic evaluations, a set of heuristics is selected, and three to five usability experts review the application or system to identify any issues that violate the set of heuristics. Usability experts identify as only SME, or they can be a "double expert." A SME is a general usability specialist who understands basic usability/UX principles and design guidelines. Double experts are usability specialists who are also an expert in the subject matter or topic under investigation (Alroobaea et al., 2014). For instance, a double expert evaluating an mHealth app might have expertise in human factors engineering as well as be a medical physician. Nielsen et al. (1994b) recommend having three to five evaluators act as participants in a heuristic evaluation, with only two or three needed if they are double experts. The evaluators assign a severity rating based on various scales (Nielsen, 1993a; Travis, 2009) so usability problems can be prioritized and addressed. UX practitioners often refer to heuristic evaluation as "expert review," and it would be considered a formal expert review because it is approached systematically, and experts evaluate against standard usability principles. Informal expert reviews, in contrast, simply involve a few usability experts reviewing a technology product for usability problems they discover on their own as opposed to adhering to same usability heuristics. Below are the typical steps to performing a traditional heuristic evaluation.

- *Step 1:* Select usability heuristics that the expert evaluators will use as a guide in their evaluation.
- *Step 2:* Identify and define priority tasks. Heuristic evaluations often look at systems as a whole, but by identifying the primary tasks that a user is more likely to perform, the heuristic evaluation can be more focused; however, this approach is sometimes referred to as heuristic walkthrough because it combines heuristics evaluation with cognitive walkthrough method, described next. Tasks are often subdivided into actions or steps or correspond to a scenario with data that evaluators use as they interact with the system.
- *Step 3:* Independent expert review. Experts independently review the system or application. There is no standard way in which evaluators can report problems. Evaluators are often asked to complete a checklist (Bright et al., 2006; Cho et al., 2022) or report usability problems on a report form, including the location in the system, a description of the issue, and screen shots (Jeffries et al., 1991). Pierotti created "Heuristic Evaluation: A System Checklist" for Xerox Corporation as a quick and easy way for evaluators to provide, "yes," "no," or "N/A" responses to a series of questions categorized under Nielsen's 10 heuristics and an additional three: skills, pleasurable and respectful interaction with the user, and privacy (Weiss, 1993). The heuristics chosen should fit the UI being evaluated and the study context. Granollers (2022) combined Nielsen's (1994b) well-known heuristics with Tognazzini's (2014) lesser-known principles of interaction design and created a checklist of 15 principles and questions to help guide usability experts' formal reviews (Granollers, 2022). Additionally, you might want to create your own set of heuristics as they are applicable to the specific UI or system you are evaluating. Lastly, the evaluators should also assign a severity rating for each potential usability problem identified. Table 8.1 lists the severity rating scale developed by Nielsen (1993a).

The severity of a usability problem is based on three factors:

o Frequency with which the problem occurs (common or rare)
o Impact of the problem on the user's ability to perform tasks and activities successfully (easy or difficult to overcome)

TABLE 8.1

Usability problem severity rating system developed by Nielsen (1993)

Severity rating	Description
0	No problem
1	Cosmetic problem—generally a problem related to the UI aesthetics
2	Minor usability problem
3	Major usability problem—major implications for the overall UX
4	Catastrophic usability problem—users are unable to achieve their goals for use or continue performing a task

    o Persistence of the problem (one-time problem that can be overcome on future encounters or will users be repeatedly bothered by the problem) (Nielsen, 1994)

- *Step 4:* Aggregate, combine, and review usability problems. The primary investigator should combine the results of all independent expert evaluators. Identical observations can be combined. Severity ratings are averaged to assign a final severity rating for each usability problem identified.

- *Step 5:* The evaluator team often meets to discuss any disagreements and reach a consensus on a final list of potential usability problems categorized by the heuristic they violate (Khajouei et al., 2017). Findings can be reported as a priority list, with recommendations and frequencies and percentages of top heuristics violated, severity rating, or location within a system might also be calculated for the purposes of identifying high-priority design flaws to be fixed or to provide a level of usability—for example, if 99 percent of the potential usability problems are assigned as a cosmetic problem, a researcher might argue that the HIT under investigation has good usability.

COGNITIVE WALKTHROUGH

Cognitive walkthrough is an expert-based usability inspection method that entails usability experts "walking through" or interacting with a system by simulating a user and performing the typical tasks a representative user is likely to perform while attempting to identify those actions or UI elements that would potentially cause usability problems (Polson et al., 1992; Wharton et al., 1994). Given that experts are simulating the typical user of the system, "the actions and feedback of the interface are compared to the user's goals and knowledge, and discrepancies between the user's expectations and the steps required by the interface are noted" (Jeffries et al., 1991). Unlike heuristic evaluations, cognitive walkthroughs take more preparation to conduct, yet may yield more fruitful insights. Cognitive walkthroughs are based on the cognitive theory of learning by exploration model (Polson & Lewis, 1990), which purports that humans integrate representations of perceptual input with background knowledge to construct a representation that will enable them to perform a task. In other words, as you explore a system, you encounter perceptual input, like buttons and icons, and associate it with existing knowledge to form an expectation of how to use the application or system to achieve goals (Polson et al., 1992). Humans also formulate expectations of how a system should respond to their interactions. The closer a system or application is to the user's mental model, the easier it will be to learn and use intuitively.

To conduct a cognitive walkthrough, you need to understand the primary user and how they will use the system, including a precise description of the system UI design, task scenarios, scope of use, and the series of actions that users take to successfully accomplish a given task (Wharton et al., 1994). Expert evaluators act like users as they attempt to perform the series of actions that are needed to accomplish each task and try to identify actions that seem to be problematic or difficult for the primary user. Like heuristic evaluations, cognitive walkthroughs are ideally completed in the early stages of the full system design lifecycle (Farzandipour et al., 2022). Following is an outline of the typical steps used in conducting a cognitive walkthrough.

- *Step 1:* Define the user and product. Describe the typical user of the product, including any characteristics or contextual aspects that may impact the user and their ability to interact with the system successfully. The more the expert evaluators know about the user, the better they will be able to "act" like a user when they walk through the system. The product or technology that will be evaluated should also be described. Technology is created for a purpose, describe what the purpose of the product or system is.
- *Step 2:* Identify the typical tasks and actions. The cognitive walkthrough involves analyzing a suite of tasks. If a system is very complex, the top five or six tasks a user performs should be listed, including the sequence of actions that should accomplish the tasks as well as a description of how the user is expected to perform the tasks before learning how to use the

system. Each task should be thoroughly described, the action sequence outlined, and the goal that users expect to achieve by performing each task stated. Additionally, task scenarios may also be used to facilitate the cognitive walkthrough, such as fictitious patient data. The tasks and actions should be documented and provided to all evaluators, so everyone is analyzing the same tasks. Take screenshots of the system during the performance of key actions and include them in the task list or, if possible, record the product walkthrough so evaluators can visualize how to perform each task. Table 8.2 illustrates an example task list for a cognitive walkthrough.

- *Step 3:* Product walkthrough by evaluators. Once the scenarios, tasks, and actions have been identified, the expert evaluators will walk through the system or application under investigation by attempting to perform each task as they simulate a primary user. A complete analysis is performed for each action identified for each task. For each action, evaluators respond to the following questions:

  1. Will the user try to achieve the right effect?
  2. Will the user notice that the correct action is available?
  3. Will the user associate the correct action with the effective they are trying to achieve?
  4. If the correct action is performed, will the user see that progress is being make toward solution of their task? (Wharton et al., 1994)

Evaluators report the following data for each task: user goals and subgoals, user actions, system responses, potential usability problems,

TABLE 8.2

Scenarios and associated tasks for cognitive walkthrough

Scenario	Tasks
Documenting treatment plan for a 12-year-old patient with influenza.	1. Select patient. 2. Enter treatment plan. 3. Submit treatment plan.
Retrieving medical record of a patient with ID 2565 who was admitted two weeks ago.	1. Search patient ID. 2. Select patient. 3. Retrieve patient history.
Archive the before and after images for a woman who has undergone cosmetic surgery.	1. Select patient. 2. Attach the images to the patient record. 3. Submit the images.

Source: Adapted from Khajouei et al. (2017).

and recommendations for how to fix the problem (Khajouei et al., 2017). Thus, the primary investigator is provided with a list of potential usability problems and descriptions, as well as screen shots if necessary. Wharton et al. (1994) suggest capturing data in multiple formats, including video-recording evaluators as they walk through the system.

- *Step 4:* Data analysis. The final step in a cognitive walkthrough is analyzing the data to create a list of potential usability problems and recommendations for how to prevent or fix each of the identified problems. Similar to a heuristic evaluation, similar usability problems may be merged and duplicates removed, and the evaluator team may meet to discuss any discrepancies and reach a consensus.

THINK-ALOUD USABILITY TEST

The think-aloud usability method is a user-based usability test and, given that real end-users are being tested, the think-aloud usability method is known as the "gold standard" of usability tests (Fonteyn et al., 1993; Marco-Ruiz et al., 2017; Nielsen et al., 1990, 1994). Think-aloud usability testing aims to go beyond just finding potential usability problems, but it is a user testing method that aims to understand users' cognitive process in HCI (Ericsson & Simon, 1980, 1984; Fonteyn et al., 1993; Lundgrén-Laine & Salanterä, 2010). The goal of UIMs is to find usability problems in the design or functionality of a system or product in order to correct them in future versions (Nielsen, 1993a; Nielsen & Landauer, 1993). Thus, the think-aloud usability test is a cognitive approach to usability testing that is best suited to assessing how easy it is for a user to carry out a task using a HIS, how well users can learn the HIS, the effects of the system on work practices, and what usability problems may occur during user interaction with the HIS (Kushniruk, 2002). During think-aloud usability tests, subjects are asked to verbalize their thoughts as they perform interactions with the artifact under investigation (Ericsson et al., 1984; Fonteyn et al., 1993; Kushniruk, 2002; Kushniruk et al., 2004). Humans' verbalization is said to reveal their cognitive behavior and information stored in their working memory so it can be tied to the task they are performing (Ericsson et al., 1993; Jones, 1989; van Someren et al., 1994).

During think-alouds, subjects are generally video- and audio-recorded in order to obtain the empirical data. The results of the subjects' verbal reports and interactions are thought to reveal the contents of the subjects' working memories and cognitive processes, which will in turn reveal the specific usability problems encountered during their interactions (Fonteyn et al., 1993; Ericsson et al., 1984; Peute et al., 2015a). Think-alouds are valuable because they uncover the "why" behind the usability problems people encounter during their interaction with technology. The combination of observational data and the verbal reports attained during think-alouds is the raw data that can be analyzed and categorized into themes of usability problems or other useful ways that enable iterative design and improvements to usability.

Concurrent versus Retrospective Think-Alouds

There are two types of think-aloud usability tests: concurrent think-alouds and retrospective think-alouds. During concurrent think-alouds, subjects are instructed to verbalize—or think aloud—their thoughts as they concurrently perform the predefined tasks and interactions with the technology under observation (Peute et al., 2015a). For instance, during a concurrent think-aloud, a subject interacting with the Teladoc website (www.teladoc.com) scrolled down the homepage when searching for the health conditions that Teladoc could treat and said, "Oh, I believe it is this down here that shows this information" (Campbell, 2020b). Retrospective think-aloud usability tests have subjects first perform the predefined tasks and activities with the technology under investigation and then retrospectively provide their verbal reports describing their interactions while watching a video-recording of their performance (Fonteyn et al., 1993; Peute et al., 2015a).

Although both methods have their limitations, concurrent think-alouds are recognized to be more effective at providing a more accurate account of subjects' cognitive processes because they are captured in real time, while the subject is performing a task, whereas retrospective studies rely on subjects' memory and ability to recall what they were thinking at the time of their interaction, which may be inconsistent or incomplete (Ericsson et al., 1984; Fonteyn et al., 1993; Lundgrén-Laine et al., 2010). Furthermore, concurrent think-alouds are verified to reveal more usability problems than retrospective think-alouds, as well as other UEMs (Cooke, 2010; Fonteyn et al., 1993; Jeffries et al., 1991; Olmsted-Hawala et al., 2010; Peute et al., 2015a, 2015b). For instance, Jeffries et al. (1991) found that more severe usability problems with user interfaces are discovered when performing think-alouds with real end-users than when performing heuristic evaluations. Similarly, Peute et al. (2015a) reported that concurrent think aloud outperformed retrospective think-alouds when evaluating the usability of a CIS. The concurrent think-alouds were demonstrated to be more effective at detecting usability issues, efficient in terms of time needed, and more valuable in terms of eliciting users' mental model of their interactions with the user interface (Peute et al., 2015a).

However, the Hawthorne effect may play a role during concurrent think-alouds, which occurs when people behave differently because they know they are being watched (Sackett Catalogue of Bias Collaboration, et al., 2017). Subjects may not verbally express why they are performing a certain action using a UI because they are trying to perform as they think the primary investigator wants them to, or they do not want to feel ashamed if they think they are performing incorrectly.

As well as soliciting more accurate verbal reports from subjects, concurrent think-alouds can be conducted in one session, whereas retrospective think-alouds require a greater time commitment from subjects because the subject must first perform the interactions, which are video- and audio-recorded, then sit and watch their recording in a second session to verbalize their thoughts. Therefore, retrospective think-alouds may require a larger or more valuable gratuity.

Below outlines the typical steps to conducting a think aloud.

- *Step 1:* Recruit representative users. Identify who are representative users of the artifact you are investigating. You will need to understand the target user group of the HIT you are investigating in order to be able to recruit participants from a sample population with similar characteristics to your target user.
- *Step 2:* Select and set-up your study context/environment. Usability tests that take place in an environment that is most representative of the user's real-life context of use will yield more accurate results. Study environments range from laboratory environments, which are artificial, to naturalistic environments where usability testing takes place in situ, which is a users' real-life context of use, such as in a clinic or an individual's home. It is recognized that usability studies that better mimic the actual environment and conditions under which a user would perform activities and tasks with the interface or system being tested yield better results (Borycki et al., 2005; Kushniruk et al., 2013).
- *Step 3:* Scenario and/or task creation. In order to have subjects interact with the technology under investigation as they would in real life, you can create scenarios, tasks, or vignettes to facilitate a simulation—for example, think-aloud usability tests that involved subjects interacting with

telemedicine websites used illness vignettes that described an illness that subjects were asked to simulate (Table 8.3) (Campbell, 2020b).

Because each telemedicine provider offered a different type of healthcare service, three separate illness vignettes were developed to enable the participant to simulate a real-life situation. When testing HIT, tasks might consist of activities such as a physician entering data into an information system or a nurse accessing online guidelines to help in the management of a patient (Kushniruk et al., 2004). In these cases, the information that physicians would enter into the system can be fabricated and reviewed by clinicians to ensure the information is an accurate representation of a patient's medical history. Likewise, the nurses might be asked to locate specific information in online guides that are intended to support their management of an artificial patient case. Alami et al. (2022) performed think-alouds with residents testing Epic Systems"'s EHR and had them perform the following pre-rounding tasks: (a) review the flow chart of

TABLE 8.3

Illness vignette used to describe the artificial testing scenario

Telemedicine provider	Illness vignette
Teladoc	You have been coughing and have had congestion in your chest for the past week. You feel extremely tired and short of breath, and often cough up clear, white mucus. You have sometimes experienced the "chills." You do not want to go any longer without feeling better, and you are afraid you might get worse if you do not see a doctor.
KADAN Institute	Since the beginning of the year, you have had an upset stomach most of the time—sometimes the pain is very severe. You often have painful cramping and extreme bloating after eating, and it doesn't go away after passing a bowel movement. Your bowel movements are inconsistent, and you are either constipated or have diarrhea. You have tried everything, from changing the foods you eat to taking Tums, but nothing seems to give you relief. You do not want to go any longer without feeling better, and you are afraid you might get worse if you do not see a doctor.
Carie Health	You have been coughing and have had congestion in your chest for the past week. You feel extremely tired and short of breath, and often cough up clear, white mucus. You have sometimes gotten the "chills." You do not want to go any longer without feeling better, and you are afraid you might get worse if you do not see a doctor.

Source: Campbell (2020b).

TABLE 8.4

Self-management tasks used during end-user testing (Or et al., 2012). The study included 11 tasks in total; only five are listed as an example

Task Number	Task Description
1	Access the blood pressure measurement module.
2	Indicate the systolic pressure value and determine whether it is normal.
3	Indicate the diastolic pressure value and determine whether it is normal
4	Access the blood glucose measurement module.
5	Select the "before breakfast" test time for blood glucose measurement.

the patient; (b) note major events that occurred over the past day; and (c) track down events that occurred overnight. End-user testing of a computer-based self-management system involved individuals who had a chronic disease performing several tasks that users of the computer-based self-management system would need to perform to effectively manage their disease using the system (Table 8.4) (Or & Tao, 2012).

• *Step 4:* Explain the study and provide examples to subjects. Prior to conducting a think-aloud, you will need to explain the study and your objectives to the participant, as well as describe how to "think aloud." Below is an excerpt from the protocol used to conduct think aloud usability tests of telemedicine websites:

"I am going to give you a scenario in which you imagine that you are sick and want to see a doctor for your condition. I will ask you to access a website and perform different activities and tasks using the website as you continue to pretend you are sick. I will ask that you talk out loud as you perform these tasks and describe your thought process and reasons why you are doing what you are doing. For example, if you want to find out information about a company, you might visit its website and click on the About button to find out more about the company. If this is the case, you will talk out loud, "I am looking for the About page to find out more about the company" (Campbell, 2020b). It is important to use the same protocol for each subject to reduce any changes to the environmental variables that may impact subjects' behaviors.

• *Step 4:* Video-/audio-record subjects' interactions. Rich qualitative data consist of both observational data and verbal reports of subjects, including the video of subjects' facial expressions and body gestures and the audio of their thoughts that they speak aloud. Being able to observe subjects' non-verbal communication simultaneous with their HCI allows researchers to make interpretations about the root cause of usability problems, as well as subjects' feelings and emotions during each interaction. Think-aloud usability tests data are known to yield rich accounts of the types of difficulties faced by users as they interact with HIT (Willis et al., 2021).

- *Step 5:* Data analysis of qualitative data using descriptive statistics and content analysis. Often, data analysis of think-aloud raw data is done using thematic analysis and inductive or deductive coding techniques. Researchers might watch the recording and code content according to an a priori coding scheme that identifies usability problems, or the usability problems may be categorized into themes as they emerge from the data. Kushniruk et al. (1996, 1997, 2004, 2005, 2008, 2013, 2015, 2016, 2019a, 2019b; Monkman et al., 2013a) have performed copious usability evaluations using cognitive-based approaches and have refined several coding schemes primarily for identifying variables such as the cognitive aspects of decision making and reasoning; usability problems stemming from socio-cognitive factors (such as limited health literacy), organizational factors (such as lack of time), or HCI factors (such as layout/organization of content and navigation); and other socio-cognitive-technical-cultural aspects of HCI that appear to stimulate usability problems in HIT. See Kushniruk et al. (2015, 2019b) for valuable codebooks. Other researchers developed original coding schemes based on inductively categorizing qualitative data from think-alouds into themes concerning challenges experienced by representative subjects when interacting with the HIT under investigation (van Osch et al., 2015; Willis et al., 2021). Qualitative data analysis software provides valuable tools used to store, manage, and analyze the type of qualitative data that is obtained from think-aloud usability studies. At the time of writing, the only tool powerful enough to allow for the coding of video- and audio-recordings as one unit (the verbal reports are able to be depicted and coded in the context of the interaction) is QSR International's NVivo 12 qualitative data analysis software. Other qualitative data analysis software products are ATLAS.ti, MAXQDA, and Dovetail.
- *Step 6:* Use findings to improve usability of HIT under investigation. The findings of think-aloud usability tests offer specific UI elements, features, and functions that can be refined to improve the usability of the HIT. Think-aloud protocol has also been used to discover other cognitive processes of individuals as they interact with HIT. For instance, Macias and Cunningham (2018) employed the think-aloud protocol to discover users' search strategies when searching for online health information.

Aitken et al. (2011) was able to discover nurses' decision-making processes regarding sedation management for critically ill patients in intensive care using think-aloud protocol alongside naturalistic observations.

HOW MANY PARTICIPANTS DO YOU NEED?

A common and critical consideration when planning a usability inspection is how many participants to recruit. There are various nuances that determine how many expert evaluators or test subjects should be recruited for each method. The popular number of "five" is based on much of the contention of Nielsen (1994a, 2000) and colleagues (Nielson & Landauer, 1993; Nielson & Molich, 1990) that only five experts or subjects are needed to discover about 80 percent of the potential usability problems in a usability inspection. When the objective is to increase the value or use of usability engineering methods, yet keep the cost to a minimum, the five-subject goal is an optimal target for both expert-based and user-based usability evaluations; however, sample sizes for each method require different considerations.

Expert-Based UIMs

For expert-based usability evaluations, a number of studies by Nielsen (1992) and colleagues (Nielson & Landauer, 1993; Nielson & Mack, 1994; Nielson & Molich, 1990) confirm that only three double experts are needed and that no more than five single experts are needed to find most of the usability problems. This is because data saturation is met by the time you have a sixth evaluator, which means that no new usability problems would be discovered by adding more evaluators. Double experts have expertise in both usability and the kind of UI being evaluated. Single experts only have expertise in usability, but may not have domain knowledge about the UI being evaluated (Nielsen, 1992). Double experts are better at finding usability problems than general usability experts, and thus only three are needed to find the majority of the usability problems (Nielsen, 1992).

User-Based UIMs

The well-known "five-users" is enough recommendation by Nielsen (1993) has been recognized as the standard number of subjects that are needed to participate in usability tests, such as think-alouds, in order to provide useful insight (Nielsen, 1993a; Virzi, 1992). Nielsen (1993a) and others (Virzi, 1992; Kushniruk, 2002) have demonstrated that testing five subjects is enough to reveal about 85 percent of the usability problems in a think-aloud usability evaluation. No new usability problems are discovered after testing five users; therefore, the "five user" rule has been standardly recognized as the most cost-effective number of representative subjects to recruit to take part in usability testing. Additionally, after each design iteration, some new usability problems may be introduced, so it is recommended that at least three rounds of usability testing be conducted with representative users. Each new group of five subjects will interact with the refined version of the product so that after about three cycles of product iterations and usability testing, the final product should have very few usability problems, and even those will likely be cosmetic in nature.

Concerns over whether five users are enough to test to be able to discover the majority of the usability problems were kindled when Faulkner (2003) demonstrated that any one random group of five subjects can discover anywhere between about 55 percent and 85 percent of the total usability problems. The idea that *every* one group of five subjects will *always* discover about 85 percent of the total usability problems is false. For instance, one set of five subjects identified only about 55 percent of the potential usability problems whereas it required about 15 subjects to identify about 90 percent of the potential usability problems (Faulkner (2003). This is because there are substantial differences in how different humans interact with technology (Egan, 1988). Faulkner's (2003) study also raised concerns about the reliability of the data obtained when testing with only five users, as well as how critical the usability problems that are missed are when testing with only five users. Other researchers agree that Faulkner's (2003) study does demonstrate that testing with more users providers greater confidence in the findings, yet the benefits of testing with more users should be weighed against the cost-savings from using a small set of subjects (van Osch et al., 2015).

Overall, UIMs should take place several times throughout the full system design lifecycle, in the formative phases, and are aimed to find and document as many usability problems in a UI as possible so that the problems can be corrected in future versions. Therefore, there is a cost-benefit ratio to consider, and testing more users—which takes time and money—to only find a few more usability problems (likely to be cosmetic) is not cost-effective. From a rigor standpoint, using as many subjects as you are able to does improve the quality of your study, but from a pragmatic standpoint, using five subjects may be sufficient in order for you to be able to discover the majority of the critical usability problems that can be addressed before the product is released. It can be argued that when conducting several iterations and rounds of usability testing throughout the full system design lifecycle, it is likely that most of the usability problems will be discovered and ameliorated by the time the product is released.

BENEFITS AND LIMITATIONS OF EXPERT-BASED AND USER-BASED USABILITY INSPECTIONS

Expert-Based Usability Inspections

Heuristic evaluations are one of the most widespread UIMs, probably because they provide a quick and easy method that can be adapted to any type of UI (Krawiec et al., 2020). Given that heuristic evaluations and cognitive walkthroughs are expert-based, they remove the additional resources that are required for recruiting and rewarding human subjects. Despite their simplicity, heuristic walkthroughs and cognitive walkthroughs are effective at finding a great number of usability problems with a UI that can be addressed before a product goes live or is made publicly available.

Studies comparing heuristic evaluations with cognitive walkthroughs demonstrate that heuristic evaluations find more potential usability issues, yet they are less severe and related to the following satisfaction usability attributes: effectiveness (ISO, 2018), efficiency, satisfaction, learnability, memorability, and errors (Khajouei et al., 2017). Even so, there was no statistically significant difference due to the number of usability problems that each method was able to uncover. Cognitive walkthroughs are able to discover more severe usability issues related to the learnability of the system or application under investigation (Khajouei et al., 2017). However, given that cognitive walkthroughs involve expert evaluators attempting to perform the primary tasks for which an end-user would use the system and simulating a representative user's behaviors while evaluating how intuitive and easy the system is to use, it is not surprising that cognitive walkthroughs are better at identifying usability problems related to learnability. Heuristic evaluations tend to evaluate the system holistically, and therefore are able to discover overall usability issues that affect user satisfaction with their overall UX. Additionally, heuristic evaluations may elicit more "false alarms," which are usability problems that the experts find, but that will not be a problem encountered by a real-life user (Jeffries, 1994). One challenge with heuristic evaluations is that they rely on evaluators' subject matter expertise to interpret the heuristics chosen and their interaction with the artifact being evaluated to identify potential usability problems. Evaluators may differ in their interpretation of a heuristic and the sheer number of design heuristics that exist can create more complexity. See Table 8.5 for a short list of usability design heuristics organized by the domain to which they are best suited.

Overall, expert-based UIMs are cheaper and faster to conduct than user-based UIMs because participants can be solicited internally and do not require a monetary reward.

TABLE 8.5

Usability principles/heuristics and domain best suited for them (listed by date of development)

Usability heuristics	No. of heuristics	Developer (reference)	Domain
Eight golden rules of interface design	8	Shneiderman (1987)	General UI interaction
Nielsen's 10 usability heuristics	10	Nielsen (1994b)	General UI interaction
Cognitive engineering principles for enhancing human–computer interaction	10	Gerhardt-Powals (1996)	General UI interaction
Laws of speech interface design	20	Weinschenk et al. (2000)	Speech/auditory UI interaction
Nielsen–Shneiderman heuristics (usability heuristics for patient medical devices)	14	Zhang et al. (2003)	Medical devices
Heuristics for health information system safety	12	Carvalho et al. (2009)	Health information systems (HIS)
Tognazzini's first principles of interaction design	19	Tognazzini (2014)	General UI interaction
Usability/health literacy heuristics for health information technology	29	Monkman & Kushniruk (2013b)	Health information systems (HIS)
Heuristic evaluation of mHealth apps (HE$_4$EH) checklist	25	Khowaja et al. (2020)	Mobile health apps (mHealth)

Although cognitive walkthrough has been demonstrated to be slightly more informative than heuristic evaluation in terms of finding realistic usability problems and critical usability problems (Khajouei et al., 2017), Polson et al. (1992) warn that cognitive walkthroughs (and any expert-based usability inspection method) are not a substitute for performing usability testing with real end-users. Cognitive walkthrough, however, is a valuable method of guiding iterative UI design by extracting claims from existing designs to inform and improve future designs (Carroll & Campbell, 1987; Gould et al., 1985).

User-Based Usability Inspections

User-based usability evaluations can arguably discover more meaningful, rich findings because they are based on the user-perspective and are therefore more representative of a real-life scenario of how the product will be used by an intended user. Thus, user-based usability tests are able to find more usability problems that are likely to occur in real life. Think-alouds, the gold standard end-user [usability] test, are rightly so because they a method to understand usability challenges in a UI from the end-user's perspective, which is what user-centered/human-centered design focuses on. Think aloud usability testing is the most effective way to find usability problems that are likely to occur in real-life. Jaspers et al. (2004) affirm that, "This approach provided a powerful way to assess clinicians' information needs, clinicians' reasoning in using the computer system and the source of their problems in using the system's interface."

When think aloud usability testing is incorporated into the full system design lifecycle as a formative method, findings can be used to improve the design of the UI or HIT prior to being implemented. For instance, iterative refinements of a UI informed by think-aloud usability testing caused a tenfold decrease in identified usability problems (Kushniruk et al., 1996, 2016; Patel & Kushniruk, 1998)

The downsides of conducting user-based usability testing include:

- *There is limited access to users.* Often, recruiting real users is difficult or recruiting a representative user group may also be challenging.
- *It is time intensive.* Usability testing with users takes more time to execute because you have to gain consent, explain the study, collect data, and make inferences as you analyze the data.

- It is costly. The data collection instruments, data analysis software, and reward you provide subjects all have a cost.

ADDITIONAL COGNITIVE APPROACHES TO USABILITY TESTING HIT

Although this chapter has discussed three of the primary methods used for conducting usability inspections, other methods to evaluate or measure usability aspects of HIT have been adapted or modified by researchers based on their study circumstances. Bhutkar et al. (2013) offer a comprehensive review of the various UIMs that have been used to evaluate HIT. Among the expert-based and user-based methods already discussed, Bhutkar et al.'s (2013) review included: task analysis; goals, operators, methods, and selection rules (GOMS) analysis; keystroke-level model (KLM); cluster analysis; and severity ratings. The last of these methods use quantitative data to measure usability or aspects of usability. More quantitative approaches to evaluating usability will be discuss in Chapter 9.

Usability testing can be conducted using various data collection instruments, such as a survey or a diary, and can be moderated or unmoderated. Generally, when collecting user insights on usability or when they encounter errors during their interaction with HIT using a survey or diary, these usability tests are considered remote and unmoderated (Campbell et al., 2021).

There are many ways to evaluate or measure usability, and a researcher's approach should take into account their study's research questions, resources, and the time available to conduct the study and perform data analysis. Generally, usability evaluations can be:

- Expert-based or user-based
- Qualitative or quantitative
- Moderated or unmoderated
- In-person or remote.

Moreover, Bhutkar et al. (2013), like other scholars (Kushniruk et al., 2002), and this book, argue that usability evaluations should take place at all stages of the full system design lifecycle, in the formative stages to test concepts or prototypes, and in the summative stages to determine whether the HIT has met usability criteria or exceeded earlier benchmarking metrics set forth in early benchmarking testing.

SUMMARY

This chapter introduced three primary, industry-standard UIMs: heuristic evaluation, cognitive walkthrough, and think aloud protocol. Heuristic evaluation and cognitive walkthrough are expert-based and are generally cheaper and quicker to facilitate, whereas think-aloud usability tests involve using representative users as subjects and require more resources. The benefit of using representative users as subjects in usability tests is that it is possible to gain richer, more accurate qualitative data as a result. However, in the full system design lifecycle, it is necessary to utilize the most suitable methods to gain the insight required and consider the resources that are available when choosing the most suitable methods. Chapter 9 will discuss several quantitative methods that are used to evaluate and measure usability, and industry-standard questionnaires that measure overall user satisfaction that are often used in combination with the qualitative usability evaluations discussed in this chapter.

9

Quantitative Usability Testing Methods and Metrics

INTRODUCTION

This chapter discusses quantitative approaches to measuring usability and usability metrics that are used to capture the extent to which certain aspects of usability are achieved. The methods discussed in this chapter include keystroke-level modeling (KLM) and eye tracking, as well as the quantitative data captured from each method. Additional usability metrics will also be presented, such as the various quantitative ways of measuring the effectiveness of a HIT under investigation (such as the number of errors made). Often quantitative data is captured during summative usability testing—after the HIT has already been implemented—to validate that the product has a sufficient level of usability or to establish benchmarking metrics for future releases or iterations of the product.

KEYSTROKE-LEVEL MODELING

KLM is an expert-based method that analyzes the time required to complete certain tasks by associating a time with the completion of a set of operations (Card et al., 1980). There is a standard set of eight operators in KLM and their execution time can be estimated from experimental data (Card et al., 1980), yet depending on the HIT being analyzed, not all eight may be used to estimate the time for a task to be completed. The eight operators are:

- K = key button press and release
- P = mouse pointing
- H = moving hands to the home position on the keyboard or to the mouse

DOI: 10.1201/9781003460886-9

- B = button press
- M = mentally preparing to perform an action
- T = typing a string of characters
- W = waiting for system to respond.

Each operator is estimated to have a fixed execution time. Summing together the execution time for each operation calculates the estimated time for a task to be completed. The KLM is designed to model an errorless execution time of routine tasks a user performs when interacting with a UI.

KLM is a quantitative technique for measuring the efficiency quality of usability that is often conducted within a mixed-methods study using the well-known HCI method, goals, operators, methods, and selection rules (GOMS) (Card et al., 1983). GOMS is a predictive model that measures procedural knowledge because it includes both the cognitive resources and the manual actions that a user must perform in order to carry out tasks on a device or system and to achieve their intended goal (Kieras, 2004). GOMs starts with a simple task analysis. Goals are what the user intends to accomplish; operators are the actions performed to achieve the goal; methods are sequences of operators that accomplish a goal; selection rules are used to identify a method in the case that multiple methods can be used to accomplish the same goal (Diaper et al, 2004). To understand the knowledge, decision-making, and cognitive processing time of a typical user of the artifact under investigation—the mental operator—researchers must perform empirical research, which is where qualitative methods may be used to understand the time a typical user requires to perform a task. Combining the human cognitive time and motor time to execute tasks offers a better understanding of the overall usability and complexity of a user interface. GOMS is an effective tool for predicting time, satisfactory performance, and task errors (Kieras, 2004).

Saitwal et al. (2010) used only seven of the operators when analyzing the Armed forces Health Longitudinal Technology Application (AHLTA) EHR system used by the U.S. military. Duncan et al. (2020) used six of those operators to explore differences in nurses' interactions with various EHRs—Cerner SurgiNet, Cerner PowerChart, Surgical Information Systems (SIS)—used at three Mayo Clinic regional campuses. See Table 9.1 for a sample KLM model of a typical task for a clinician interacting with an EHR.

Any deviation from the "happy path" or typical sequence of actions that the user should perform to complete a task is considered an error, and allows investigators to identify specific tasks that are problematic.

TABLE 9.1

Sample KLM for the task of "locating the patient" in an EHR

Step/action	Description	Operator	Time (seconds)
1	Think of location in main menu.	M	1.2
2	Extend hand towards mouse.	H	0.4
3	Extend the mouse to Go in main menu.	P	1.1
4	Enter patient's name in search bar.	T	2.6
5	Extend the mouse to the located patient name.	P	1.1
6	Click on the name of the patient.	B	0.1
Return with goal accomplished		**Total**	6.5

Source: Modified from Saitwal et al. (2010).

When combined with empirical research, KLMs are useful for determining what percentage of total mental operators are due to the design of the interface and how they could be reduced or eliminated (Saitwal et al., 2010). KLMs can also be used to determine benchmarking metrics for tasks and tested after a redesign of the UI, which was intended to improve the workflow or efficiency of tasks to be completed.

USABILITY METRICS

Different qualities or attributes of usability are often captured during mixed-methods as quantitative data. Usability metrics reveal aspects of the user inter-action that are tied to effectiveness, efficiency, or satisfaction, and that are observable and can be counted in some way (González et al., 2009). Aspects of usability that are influenced by user preferences or attitudes and not tied to the actual interaction with the UI, but more reflective of the actual UX, are not considered usability metrics. Usability metrics serve as additional data to be able to triangulate with other data collected and can corroborate other quantitative or qualitative results or spur the need to investigate further. Quantitative usability metrics can act as predictive measures and increase the validity of a study (the extent to which it measures what it claims to measure) or benchmarking metrics for a future iteration of the HIT to be tested against. Studies that intend to use usability metrics as benchmarking metrics with the goal of comparing against future iterations must first develop the usability objectives, then determine whether the product under investigation has met these objectives (Lewis, 2006).

Studies that use a large population of representative users can also use quantitative results of user performance as a metric of generalizability (Polit & Beck, 2010). For instance, Campbell et al. (2021) used a large, heterogeneous sample population of representative users to test whether telemedicine platforms were usable by the general public for which they were intended. Results were that 95 per cent of the participants in the remote usability testing session of the Teladoc website (prior to a redesign) were able to complete all tasks successfully (Campbell et al., 2021) This finding can be generalized to the larger public for whom Teladoc is offered, and it can be suggested that the larger public would also be able to use the Teladoc successfully.

Hornbæk (2006) performed a survey of current practices in usability studies over the entire HCI landscape and reported similar challenges (as discussed in Chapters 2 and 3) with measuring usability in practice, including the challenges posed by the pluralistic definition of usability when trying to standardize attributes and metrics; that usability cannot be directly measured because it is a composite of subjective (human-based) and contextual (environmental-based) factors; and approaches to user-centered design and usability depending on how one measures usability and the resources available to do so. Hornbæk (2006) effectively defined each usability attribute (effectiveness, efficiency, and user satisfaction) and reported on the ways scholars have attempted to measure each of these attributes and the type of quantitative data collected.

Most of the HCI community (González et al., 2009; Hornbæk, 2006; Yen et al., 2012), including the U.S. National Institute of Standards and Technology (Lowry et al., 2012), adhere to the definitions offered by the ISO (2018) in ISO 9241:

- Effectiveness is the accuracy and completion with which a user is able to achieve their goals for use.
- Efficiency refers to the resources expended in relation to the accuracy and completeness with which users achieve goals.
- Satisfaction is the degree to which the user is happy with their experience or expresses a positive attitude towards the product they interacted with. (González et al., 2009; Hornbæk, 2006; ISO, 2018; Yen et al., 2012)

Similarly, Wronikowska et al. (2021) performed a systematic review of usability studies of EHRs to understand the "breadth of usability evaluation methods, metrics, and associated measurement techniques" applied in the study of EHRs and further evaluated metrics associated with "learnability," "memorability," and "errors" components. Wronikowska et al.'s (2021) systematic review revealed that not much has changed in terms of how usability is measured and the challenges with evaluating usability, especially in the healthcare field.

How to measure usability is an important question in HCI research, and in being able to predict the impact of HIT on users. For instance, computerized physician order entry (CPOE) systems, which are usually integrated with clinical decision support systems (CDS), were originally developed to improve the safety of medication orders by offering clinicians preferred drugs, doses, and dispensing information, as well as alerting clinicians about patient allergies or interactions with other drugs. CPOE, if usable, can act as an error-prevention tool and reduce medication errors and adverse drug reactions in hospitals (Alotaibi et al., 2017; Devine et al., 2010). However, implementing features like "hard stops" in CPOEs can have negative consequences on patients' time-to-treatment, resulting in clinically significant treatment delays (Powers et al., 2018). "Hard stop" alerts are those that prevent a clinician from taking action and are implemented in CPOEs and CDSs to attenuate clinicians' tendency to ignore repeated alerts. Evaluating the usability of CPOEs and discovering the usability of various alert types is critical for understanding how to design HIT that will be used successfully in the healthcare context in the way it is intended to be delivered and that will have positive outcomes.

A list of common usability metrics has been synthesized from several studies, with the metrics categorized as a usability metric of efficiency, effectiveness, or user satisfaction (Dumas et al., 1999; Hornbæk, 2006; Wronikowska et al., 2021) and listed in Table 9.2. Keep in mind that usability is a dynamic and multifaceted construct, and that usability metrics are interrelated so the measurement techniques or data collection instruments used are often able to capture multiple usability metrics.

Quantitative usability data is frequently captured automatically within the HIT under investigation and collected and analyzed alongside other data, such as in Khairat et al.'s (2020, 2021) two studies. In one study, Khairat et al. (2021) compared individual user EHR activity data, such as time in the system and time spent taking notes, which was captured in the Epic EHR (Epic Systems'), between physician type among general and specialty pediatricians. In a mixed-methods study evaluating the association between EHR use and physician fatigue, the following usability metrics were collected: task completion times, number of mouse clicks, and number of screens visited (Khairat et al., 2020). These usability metrics were compared with each participant's psychological fatigue level, which was measured using eye tracking glasses (Tobii Pro Glasses 2) by pupillometry (changes in pupil size with lower scores indicating greater fatigue) (Khairat et al., 2020).

TABLE 9.2

Usability metrics and data collection methods

Usability component	Usability metric	Description	Measurements
Effectiveness	Task completion success	Measures whether users are able to complete tasks or not	• Number of correct tasks users complete (or correct responses) • Number of tasks users failed to complete within a set time • Number of tasks users gave up and failed to complete • Number/percentage of users who successfully completed tasks
	Accuracy	Measures the number of errors users make	• Number of errors users make during the process of completing tasks • Number of errors users make minus the number of hints an experimenter gives • Spatial accuracy, measured as the distance to a target from the position indicated by the user • Precision accuracy, measured by the ratio of the number of correct documents retrieved to the total number of documents retrieved
	Recall	Measures how much information users can recall after interacting with a UI	• Number of information pieces or amount of content users are able to recall
	Completeness	Measures the extent to which tasks are solved (in cases where it does not make sense to suggest that users made errors, but reached solutions of different levels of completeness)	• Number of clicks to complete a task • Number of secondary tasks solved • Proportion of relevant information pieces or content found in information-retrieval tasks
	Quality of outcome	Measures the outcome of tasks (outcome measured depends on the task and should be determined by the primary research objectives and purpose of the artifact under investigation)	• Level or depth of understanding using tests • Quality of content using a five-point grading scale • Involvement and engagement users express when completing tasks scored by judges using a three-point rating scale • Users' ability to predict an event or variable

Efficiency		
Task completion time	Measures how long users take to complete tasks	• Total time to complete a tasks • Time taken to complete certain parts of a task • Times in between certain actions
Input rate	Measures the time take for users to enter or input information or data	• Text entry speed (words per minute) • Corrected text entry speed (words per minute)
Mental/cognitive effort	Measures the cognitive resources users spend to complete tasks or during an interaction	• NASA's Task Load Index • Heart rate variability • Subjective time estimates
Usage patterns	Measures how the interface is used	• Number of times a certain feature is interacted with or action is performed • Number of keystrokes used for completing data entry tasks • Number of mouse clicks used to complete tasks • How much information users access or retrieve to complete certain tasks • Deviations from optimal solution or "happy path" to complete a task • Ratio of actual distance traveled to shortest distance traveled • Number of target entries into a specific region, leaving, and re-entering
Communication effort	Measures the resources users expend in communication	• Number of turns in group conversation • Number of grounding questions asked between members in a cooperative effort
Learning	Measures changes in efficiency as an indicator of learning	• Time needed to complete tasks (over several sessions) • Reading rate (words per minute) • Expert assessment of task completion ease

(*continued*)

TABLE 9.2 (Continued)

Usability metrics and data collection methods

Usability component	Usability metric	Description	Measurements
User satisfaction	Overall user satisfaction	Measures users' attitude, sentiment, or emotional state during or after their interaction with the artifact under investigation (ease-of-use and usefulness are often constructs remarked on while capturing the overall user satisfaction data)	• Standardized questionnaires are research instruments used for collecting data about a user's experience. They measure and quantify user satisfaction. Common scales include: Questionnaire for User Interface Satisfaction (QUIS) and System Usability Scale (SUS). • General user comments or feedback related to their interaction (either positive or negative)
	Preference	Measures which interface users prefer using	• Selection of UI preferred • Rank ordering a series of UI according to most preferred to least preferred best or like least
	Specific attitudes	Measures of a specific attitude towards or perception of a UI	• Ranking or selection of a point that best represents their response to a question using a Likert scale
	Perception of outcomes	Measures users' rating of their perception of the outcomes of the interaction	• Ranking or selection of a point that best represents their response to a question using a Likert scale
	Perception of interaction	Measures users' rating of their perception of the process of interaction	• Ranking or selection of a point that best represents their response to a question using a Likert scale

Source: Dumas et al. (1999); Hornbæk (2006); Wronikowska et al. (2021).

To reiterate, usability metrics should be determined based on how one defines usability and the research objectives. For instance, Woodruff et al. (2001) counted the number of pages a subject visited when testing three different versions of thumbnails as they established the number of pages as a quality-in-use metric. Increased pages visited indicated better usability. Yet, in other studies, the more pages a user visits might indicate poorer usability if testing the navigation or users' ability to find specific information they are asked to find. There are myriad standardized user satisfaction questionnaires that attempt to gauge and quantify the user experience; these will be discussed in Chapter 10.

EYE-TRACKING

Eye-tracking is a quantitative approach to tracking and monitoring users' visual attention and interactions with a webpage or UI, including the locations on which their eyes focus and the path their eyes take when scrolling, scanning, reading, and navigating a UI. Because humans' eyes naturally and automatically move to maintain or shift attention between visual areas, eye-tracking devices are able to capture various quantitative data (Goldberg & Wichansky, 2003). Eye-tracking measures how long and how often a user looks at particular areas of interest (AOI) and the length and speed of eye movements (Ooms et al., 2015; Visweswaran et al., 2021). Key metrics that are captured from eye-tracking data include fixations and saccades (Asan & Yang, 2015; Doberne et al., 2015), among other fixation and eye movement-related measures that can be captured with eye-tracking devices.

The position where the eyes focus—the point of regard (POR) on a screen or UI—is typically expressed using pixels, which are screen coordinates. Following is a short list of common eye-tracking metrics and a definition:

- Fixation: a moment (typically longer than longer than 300 milliseconds) in which the eyes are relatively stationary.
- Saccade: rapid eye movement between fixations, typically lasing for 20–35 seconds.
- Fixation duration: length, in time, of a fixation.
- Fixation count: number of fixations.
- Dwell time: the accumulated length of time the eyes fixate on a certain AOI or piece of content, such as words or passages of text.

- Scan-path or gaze-path: the path a participant's eyes take while scanning the visual information or UI; a complete sequence of fixations and interconnecting saccades (Asan et al., 2015; Champlin et al., 2021; Djamasbi et al., 2007; Ooms et al., 2015; Poole & Ball, 2006; Roche et al., 2022).

Eye fixations and movements have been associated with different forms of cognitive information processing and behaviors, such as the difficulty of understanding particular pieces of information or decision-making processes. For instance, high fixation rates are demonstrated to indicate a user has a strong level of interest in an AOI (Velazquez & Pasch, 2014), whereas longer fixation rates on an AOI indicate users have difficulty processing that information (Jacob & Karn, 2003). Many successive fixations in a short duration have been associated with inefficient visual search (Goldberg, 2000). Saccades are instigated when a critical cognitive event occurs and represents a swift attention shift (Yang & McConkie, 2001).

Eye-tracking is often conducted in correspondence with another primary qualitative method because eye-tracking data reveals "what" users do, but not "why." Additionally, eye-tracking data is valuable for methodological triangulation because it offers a quantitative data set that can be compared with and interpreted alongside other quantitative or qualitative data (Champlin et al., 2021). Therefore, many studies pair eye-tracking studies with log-file metrics, interviews, or think-aloud usability testing with representative users. For instance, both Khairat et al. (2021) and Nelson et al. (2015) used eye-tracking metrics to discover the time on task, screens used, and AOIs on which physicians and pharmacists focused, mostly in EHRs to help inform the design of EHR that supported physicians' and pharmacists' workflow and the presentation of information they used to made medical and prescription decisions.

Areas of interest (AOI) are generally established at the start of a study as areas of a UI on which a researcher wants to focus. Three AOIs were identified as task-related regions at the start of a study that sought to understand surgeons' main fixation points in order to improve the design of a surgical interface for kidney tumor cryoablation (Erol Barkana & Açık, 2014). Upon analysis of the participants' fixations, saccades, and dwell time during their interaction with the surgical interface, it was discovered that participants concentrated on informative areas of the UI where the number of Computer Tomography (CT) images was reduced, thereby reducing their cognitive load (Erol Barkana et al., 2014).

Various companies manufacture the technology required to collect and analyze eye-tracking data. Generally, eye-tracking technology is sold as an "eye-tracking system," and one must invest in the eye-tracker and analysis software. Tobii and Gazepoint are two popular eye-tracking technology companies that have mounted and wearable (mobile eye-tracking glasses) available. In addition to collecting the quantitative eye-tracking data that measure fixations and saccades in seconds, heat maps and gaze plots are two data visuals that can be produced and analyzed using the eye-tracking method. Heat maps illustrate the various areas that are given attention on a UI or screen by using a gradient of colors—usually green to red—where green areas represent less-attended areas and red areas represent highly attended areas (the areas on the UI on which participants focused most). Gaze plots illustrate the location of eye movements during a participant's interaction with the UI or visual information. See Figure 9.1 for an example of a heat map and gaze plot produced in Champlin et al.'s (2021) study.

Considering the multidimensional nature of eye-tracking data that can be captured and analyzed, as well as how eye-tracking metrics have been associated with various human cognitive processing capabilities and user behaviors, it is difficult to compare the findings across eye-tracking studies in the healthcare space, yet eye-tracking is increasingly becoming a secondary quantitative method employed in mixed-method usability studies. Eghdam et al. (2011) leveraged eye-tracking data to explore physicians' use of an antibiotic support visualization. Doberne et al. (2015) employed eye-tracking in a mixed-methods usability study of a EHR to characterize the typical workflow patterns and

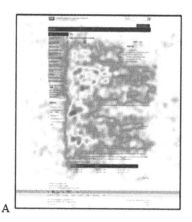
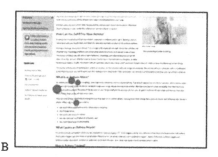

FIGURE 9.1

Heat map (A) and gaze plot (B) of low health literacy hearing participants viewing online health information produced using Tobii Pro X3 eye-tracking glasses and Tobii Studio software.

Source: **Champlin et al. (2021).**

screens used by physicians. Henneman et al. (2008) discovered that the majority of medical provider participants do not verify patient identification information by collecting and analyzing eye-tracking data. Roche et al. (2022) used fixations on previously established areas of interest (AOIs) on a patient monitor to measure anesthesia providers' patient monitoring during critical and non-critical situations, as well as analyzing these metrics against the experience level of the participants. Anesthesia providers increased their visual attention to the patient monitor during critical situations, yet focused on only a few vital signs (Roche et al., 2022). Because eye-tracking metrics have been associated with various human cognitive processing behaviors, such as search, comprehension, judgement, and decision-making, implementing eye-tracking in a mixed-method usability study of HIT is a valuable and robust way to approach evaluating HIT usability.

USABILITY IN CONTEXT

Context is significant when determining usability, as each aspect of usability is influenced by context of use, as well as subjective factors, such as physical and cognitive capabilities and emotional state. Because usability is influenced by a variety of factors, quantitative methods are usually secondary to qualitative research in usability studies and quantitative results must be considered in light of these other influencers of usability. Choudhury et al. (2022) set out to test these individual and contextual mediators of usability of patient portals and used both a large sample of representative users of the U.S. general public and the well-known U.S.-based Health Information National Trends Survey (HINTS) to discover whether patients' understanding of patient portals and/or their mental health status impacted their perception of the quality of care. Choudhury et al. (2022) discovered that patients' ability to use patient portals and understand their medical information positively influenced their perception of the quality of care. In addition, patients who experienced health conditions—most notably heart problems—suffered negative mental health implications, which also influenced their perception of quality of care. This research highlights the association between individual and contextual determinants of usability and how they cannot be considered independent variables of usability, but must always be interpreted and presented in the light of the context of use and subjective factors.

The findings show the importance of comprehension of displayed online medical information and how the patient-centered design of patient portals can help health care systems improve patients' overall care perception, which potentially helps retain patients in their systems. The study also highlights the importance of considering potential users' attributes such as age, existing ailments, and various mental health statuses during the patient portal design process.

(Choudhury et al., 2022)

How Many Participants Do You Need for Quantitative Studies?

The general consensus is that the larger the sample size, the more reliable and generalizable your study's results will be (Cohen, 1988). Increasing the effectiveness of usability studies is a major aim of HCI researchers, yet it is important to consider that quantitative results are merely secondary to qualitative findings because they cannot tell you why users act as they do when interacting with a UI nor how to fix usability problems that are caused by a design flaw. Quantitative findings can be used to corroborate your conclusions or be used as established benchmarks for future usability testing of refined and enhanced versions of a UI. Another consideration is feasibility of your methods:

- How much time do you have to recruit a large sample population of representative users?
- How difficult is it for you to recruit the target user you are seeking for your study?
- How much gratuity are you able to give?
- How much value does the quantitative findings add to your study and achieving your study's objectives?

Alroobaea et al. (2014) provide some quick numbers for how many participants you should recruit for common quantitative usability studies to be considered relatively rigorous:

- General usability/user testing: 20 users
- Card sorting: 15 users
- Eye-tracking: 39 users.

Although Alroobaea et al. (2014) provide some good numbers to support how many participants should be recruited to achieve a level of rigor, your research questions and resources available to perform your study are more important for informing your study design and recruitment efforts.

SUMMARY

This chapter discussed common quantitative approaches to evaluating and measuring the usability of HIT. KLM is a method used to understand the length of time users take to complete tasks and eye-tracking is a method to understand the location and movement of users' eyes as they interact with a UI. Both approaches capture quantitative data that can be analyzed and interpreted in various ways to allow a researcher to triangulate them with other data collected. Various usability components, such as efficiency or effectiveness, can also be quantified and captured from log-files (from the HIT) or timers during usability testing sessions. Quantitative usability methods are typically conducted at the end of a full system design lifecycle, either just before or just after implementation, and are often the secondary method included in mixed-methods studies. The purpose of summative UX methods is to provide additional support that a design is usable, to generalize to the target population, and to capture benchmarking metrics to be tested against in future UX research. Chapter 10 will offer several standardized questionnaires that are often used as another quantitative approach to measuring the usability and UX of HIT.

10

Post-Study Surveys and Retrospective Questionnaires

INTRODUCTION

This chapter discusses several standardized surveys and questionnaires that quantitatively measure usability/UX or certain aspects of the UX. The most popular standardized scale that will be discussed is the System Usability Scale (SUS), as it is the most leveraged assessment of usability across all disciplines and industry spaces. Several other common questionnaires that are used to evaluate usability, user satisfaction, acceptance, or other UX aspects will be introduced, including the Post-Study System Usability Questionnaire (PSSUQ), the Telemedicine Satisfaction and Usefulness Questionnaire (TSUQ), the Questionnaire for User Interface Satisfaction (QUIS), and the NASA-Task Load Index (NASA-TLX). The chapter will conclude with a brief explanation of why and how these standardized scales should be used and modified based on one's study parameters.

WHY USE POST-STUDY DATA-COLLECTION INSTRUMENTS?

Employing a post-study survey or questionnaire is a fairly simple and quick method to collecting additional end-user data, which becomes another data set that contributes to a comprehensive mixed-methods study. Numerous researchers consider implementing post-usability test or retrospective surveys and questionnaires to be a valuable addition to a mixed-methods study of HIT and other user interfaces, as well as an integral part of the iterative, user-centered design process (Johnson et al., 2005; Kushniruk et al., 1997; Kushniruk et al.,

DOI: 10.1201/9781003460886-10

2001; Kushniruk et al., 2013). When applied immediately following subjects' interaction with a technology being tested, retrospective questionnaires allow for a deeper understanding of the user experience and subjective impression of the system's usability because subjects are less prone to have recall problems regarding their experience (Kushniruk et al., 1997, 2001, 2013, 2019a). There is also evidence supporting the assertation that when questionnaires are implemented retrospectively, they afford valuable predictive data that can be applied directly to the iterative design or user-centered design of HIS and user interfaces advocated by numerous scholars (Horsky et al., 2016; Johnson et al., 2005; Kushniruk et al., 1997, 2001, 2002, 2004; Wolpin et al., 2015). Survey and questionnaire results afford data triangulation, which can either corroborate or contradict other data obtained in a mixed-methods study. If used as a single method, traditional survey and questionnaire data only inform researchers about what users say they would do using a HIT—it measures only their perception of how they would behave. However, what people say they will do is often considerably different from their actual behavior, which is why usability testing is a critical component of full system design lifecycle (Eysenbach et al., 2002; Kushniruk et al., 1996). Retrospective questionnaires can also solicit additional specific user feedback about their experience interacting with a HIT, which can be better assessed after a user has had the experience. Specific questions can be developed that ask users to suggest specific, concrete ways to improve their experience or the usability of the HIT with which they interacted. These findings can be applied directly to iterations in the design of HIT. The SUS, described first, will be the only usability scale discussed in detail; the others presented subsequently will be introduced briefly, given the sheer number of post-study questionnaires that have been developed to measure various aspects of the user interaction. The decision to implement a post-study questionnaire and which questionnaire to select should be based on a study's research objectives and what construct or aspect of the user interaction one wants to measure.

WHY USE PSYCHOMETRICALLY TESTED QUESTIONNAIRES TO MEASURE USABILITY OR RELATED ASPECTS?

The questionnaires and surveys discussed in this chapter are often appended at the end of a study; however, they can also be applied as a standalone study because they provide a foundation for understanding the usability of HIT and can often be compared with other similar HIT in the market. For instance, the System Usability Scale (SUS) is ideal for comparing a system's overall usability to other systems, as it is the most reliable and validated usability scale among the many proprietary questionnaires that exist (Sauro, 2011), and is cited in more than 1200 publications and translated in eight languages (Sousa et al., 2017). Additionally, a single study of telemedicine can use the Telemedicine Usability Questionnaire (TUQ) to compare patients' perceptions of usability against physicians' perceptions of usability because both user groups must find telemedicine to have a sufficient level of usability to be adopted and utilized successfully when implemented (Parmanto et al., 2016). Thus, the standardized scales discussed in this chapter can be implemented post-study or as a standalone study to collect end-user feedback about the usability of a technology and other aspects of their UX. The questionnaires and surveys are categorized as system-agnostic for those that can be applied to any technology or system, and HIT-specific for those that were developed for eHealth, mHealth, and other heath- and healthcare-related technology; additional questionnaires and surveys are presented that focus on a single attribute or implementation, such as cognitive load.

SYSTEM-AGNOSTIC

System Usability Scale (SUS)

The System Usability Scale (SUS) is a 10-item Likert scale that measures users' subjective perceptions of usability following their interaction with a technology or system. See the SUS in Table 10.1.

The SUS was developed by John Brooke in 1986, as part of the usability engineering program at Digital Equipment Co Ltd (Reading, United Kingdom), after seeing an industry need for a tool that could quickly assess a user's subjective rating of a product's usability and be widely applied across different applications, websites, systems, and domains (Brooke, 2013). Since its development, the SUS has been widely adopted across industries and validated in many studies so it affords the ability to compare the "perceived usability" of different artifacts because of its standardization and shared scoring values (Lewis & Sauro, 2009, 2018). The popularity of the SUS for evaluating HIT usability and overall subjective user satisfaction is understandable given the many benefits:

TABLE 10.1

The SUS asks respondents to indicate their degree of agreement or disagreement with a statement regarding a system's usability (brooke, 1986) using a five-point likert scale with 1 = Strongly disagree and 5 = Strongly agree

Statement	1 Strongly disagree	2 Disagree	3 Neither agree nor disagree	4 Agree	5 Strongly agree
1 I think that I would like to use this system frequently.					
2 I found the system unnecessarily complex.					
3 I thought the system was easy to use.					
4 I think that I would need the support of a technical person to be able to use this system.					
5 I found the various functions in this system were well integrated.					
6 I thought there was too much inconsistency in this system.					
7 I would imagine that most people would learn to use this system very quickly.					
8 I found the system very cumbersome to use.					
9 I felt very confident using the system.					
10 I needed to learn a lot of things before I could get going with this system.					

Please indicate your level of agreement or disagreement with the following statements about your experience interacting with the system using the five-point Likert scale.

- *Validation.* The construct validity and overall reliability as a quantitative metric of usability has been well-validated across numerous studies (Bangor et al, 2009; Georgsson et al., 2016; Lewis, 2006; Li et al., 2013; Sauro & Lewis, 2009).

- *Implementation.* It is easy to implement retrospectively to a study or as a single method alone by developing it into a survey platform or by handing out a hard copy for participants to complete.
- *Length.* It consists of just 10 easy-to-understand questions.
- *Interpretation.* There are many ways to interpret the scores that can be meaningfully presented to different audiences.
- *Cost-effectiveness.* It is freely available in Brooke's (1986) article, from many online sources, and in Appendix B of this book.

The SUS is the most frequently used quantitative usability measurement instrument in the healthcare space with references in numerous studies (Broekhuis et al., 2019; Farrahi et al., 2019; Georgsson et al., 2016; Khairat et al., 2019; Murray-Torres et al., 2019; Richardson et al, 2017; Wronikowska et al., 2021). The SUS provides a single metric that gauges users' overall impression of the usability of a system and there are many ways to interpret SUS scores. It is important to remember that the SUS score does not divulge any one dimension of usability. Brooke (2013) warns that the individual statements do not diagnose specific features or functions of the system that lead to unsatisfactory use by the end-user.

How to Score the SUS

To score an SUS, you first have to transform all individual item scores into a shared scoring system, from 0–4. Follow these steps:

1. For all odd items (all positive statements: 1, 3, 5, 7, 9), subtract one point from the user's response. Example: 4 – 1 = 3.
2. For all even items (all negative statements: 2, 4, 6, 8, 10) subtract the user's response from five. Example: 5 – 5 = 0
3. Add up the converted values to calculate a total score ranging from 0 to 40.
4. Finally, convert the total score into a value ranging from 0 to 100 by multiplying by 2.5. Example: 22 * 2.5 = 55.

How to Interpret the SUS Score

The final SUS score is based on a scale of 0–100, which is a percentile ranking of any one subject's overall perceived usability of the system (Brooke, 1986;

Sauro, 2011, 2019). According to research, the average SUS score is 68, which is considered to be above average (Brooke, 2013; Sauro, 2011). The percentile ranking of the original SUS score is similar to grading on a curve with which academics might be familiar (Lewis et al., 2018; Sauro, 2011). Therefore, the mean score of 68 is in the 50th percentile is equivalent to a "C" letter grade. A score above 80.3 gets an "A" for usability and any score below 51 is considered to have very poor usability and is assigned an "F" letter grade (Lewis et al., 2018; Sauro 2011, 2019). Because the SUS is known to be easy to administer in practice, and also valid and reliable, other scholars have developed alternative means to interpret the SUS score (Bangor et al., 2009; Sauro, 2018) that are more effective at illustrating the overall usability of the system.

Along with the curved grading scale, Bangor et al. (2009) developed an adjective that expresses subjects' sentiment when using the technology being evaluated to align with each percentile ranking and grade to support a better understanding of users' perceived usability of the system. Several usability and UX experts have rounded these scores to ease interpretation of the overall usability and converted them into the letter grade and adjective rating that Bangor et al. (2009) added to the SUS scale ranking (Alathas, 2018; Lewis et al., 2018; T.W., (n.d.). Table 10.2 offers a general guideline for interpreting the SUS; however, more granular interpretive options are defined by Bangor et al. (2009); Lewis et al. (2018); and Sauro (2018).

Decades' worth of research demonstrates that the SUS is an effective, reliable, and valid tool for measuring the usability of a system or technology from the user's perspective and that it performs similarly when using a large sample population or as few as eight to 12 end-users (Bangor et al., 2009; Sauro, 2011; Tullis & Stetson, 2004).

TABLE 10.2

Various SUS score interpretations including the SUS score, percentile range, letter grade, and adjective

SUS Score	Percentile range	Grade	Adjective rating
> 80.3	Top 15 percentile	A	Excellent
68–80.3	50–85 percentiles	B	Good
68	50th percentile (medium)	C	Okay
51–68	15–50	D	Poor
< 51	Bottom 15 percentile	F	Awful

The SUS is system agnostic and is freely available via many online sources (Sauro, 2011, 2018).

Post-Study System Usability Questionnaire (PSSUQ)

The Post-Study System Usability Questionnaire (PSSUQ) is similar to the SUS in that it assesses users' perceptions of a system's usability and user satisfaction; however, it was developed by Lewis (1992) specifically to be implemented as a post-usability test questionnaire for scenario-based usability studies. The PSSUQ is based on a seven-point Likert scale and consists of 18 questions (in the original version—see Table 10.2) pertaining specifically to scenario-based usability studies that have subjects perform specific tasks and activities while interacting with a technology (Lewis, 1992). The PSSUQ asks participants to respond with their level of agreement or disagreement with statements phrased in the past tense, referencing tasks they have just completed.

The PSSUQ results can be categorized in three domains: the system's ease of use and efficiency in performing tasks, information quality, and interface quality (van Osch et al., 2015). Higher scores indicate higher usability. Note that the original scale used a Likert scale with "1" equaling "strongly agree," thus lower scores indicated higher usability, but newer versions of the PSSUQ use the seven-point Likert scale for agreement with "1" equaling "strongly disagree." Since its development, the PSSUQ has been modified several times to include or exclude some items, yet the PSSUQ remains a highly reliable scale to use to measure overall system usability from the user's perspective (Lewis, 2002). The PSSUQ is system agnostic and is freely available via many online sources (Sauro, 2019).

Questionnaire for User Interface Satisfaction (QUIS)

The Questionnaire for User Interface Satisfaction (QUIS) is a measurement tool developed by Chin et al. (1988) to measure the satisfaction of users with their interaction with a computer interface. QUIS consists of 27 items in five sections (Chin, 1988). The first section measures the overall satisfaction, and the four others measure user satisfaction regarding screen, terminology and information, learning, and system capabilities (Hajesmaeel-Gohari & Bahaadinbeigy, 2021). The QUIS is not freely available, as it is copyrighted and trademark protected by the University of Maryland (University of Maryland UM Ventures).

TABLE 10.3

The PSSUQ asks respondents to read each statement and indicate how strongly they agree or disagree with each statement using a seven-point likert scale where 1 = Strongly disagree and 7 = Strongly agree

	Statement	1 Strongly disagree	2 Disagree	3 Somewhat disagree	4 Neither agree nor disagree	5 Somewhat agree	6 Agree	7 Strongly agree
1	The system has all the functions and capabilities I expect it to have.							
2	Overall, I am satisfied with this system.							
3	Overall, I am satisfied with how easy it is to use this system.							
4	It was simple to use this system.							
5	I could effectively complete the tasks and scenarios using this system.							
6	I was able to complete the tasks and scenarios quickly using this system.							
7	I was able to efficiently complete the tasks and scenarios using this system.							
8	I felt comfortable using this system.							
9	It was easy to learn to use this system.							
10	The interface of this system was pleasant.							
11	I liked using the interface of this system.							
12	The organization of information on the system screens was clear.							
13	The system gave error messages that clearly told me how to fix problems.							
14	Whenever I made a mistake using the system, I could recover quickly and easily.							
15	The information provided with this system (online help, documentation) was clear.							
16	It was easy to find the information I needed.							
17	The information provided for the system was easy to understand.							
18	The information was effective in heling me complete the tasks and scenarios.							

Please read each statement and indicate how strongly you agree or disagree with each statement.

Source: Lewis (1992).

USABILITY METRIC FOR USER EXPERIENCE (UMUX)

The Usability Metric for User Experience (UMUX) is a four-item Likert scale that provides a subjective metric of a system's usability. UMUX is comparable to the SUS; however, it is shorter than the SUS and may be easier to implement in some study contexts. The UMUX can be administered as a post-study questionnaire or as a standalone survey (Finstad, 2010).

HEALTH INFORMATION TECHNOLOGY (HIT)-SPECIFIC

Health Information Technology Usability Evaluation Scale (Health-ITUES)

Brown et al. (2013) developed the Health Information Technology Usability Evaluation Scale (Health-ITUES) specifically to evaluate the usability of mHealth technology, such as mobile health apps. The Health-ITUES integrates concepts from the technology acceptance model (TAM), the ISO 9241-11 definition of usability, and Nielsen's (1994), Shneiderman et al.'s (2010), and Norman's (2013) usability principles. It covers error prevention; completeness; memorability; information needs; flexibility/customizability; learnability; performance speed; competency; and other outcomes. The Health-ITUES has demonstrated appropriateness usefulness in the evaluation mHealth technology (Schnall et al., 2018).

Patient Assessment of Communication During Telemedicine (PACT) Questionnaire

The Patient Assessment of Communication During Telemedicine (PACT) is a 33-item self-report data collection instrument that assesses patients' perceptions of the communication between a physician during a telemedicine interaction (Agha et al., 2009). The PACT contains items that measure patient satisfaction with the communication style of the physician, as well as convenience, privacy, technical quality, and overall quality of the telemedicine visit (Agha et al., 2009). Items are rated on a five-point Likert scale ranging from "Not at all" to "Very much." Higher scores reflect higher satisfaction.

Perceived Telemedicine Importance, Disadvantages, and Barriers (PTIDB)

The Perceived Telemedicine Importance, Disadvantages, and Barriers (PTIDB) is a survey developed to assess healthcare professionals' perceptions of telemedicine in order to identify barriers to implementation and success that can be used to inform the decision-making of policymakers (Youssef et al., 2022). The PTIDB consists of 24 questions under four domains: importance of using telemedicine; disadvantages of telemedicine technology; advantages of using telemedicine; and barriers to utilizing telemedicine. The PTIDB uses a five-point Likert scale ranging from "strongly disagree" to "strongly agree." Although the PTIDB was developed to be deployed in Egypt, it has important applications in all geographic areas since telemedicine is such an important component of the healthcare system. The PTIDB is one way to assess the success of telemedicine implementation.

Telehealth Usability Questionnaire (TUQ)

The Telehealth Usability Questionnaire (TUQ) is one of the most popular instruments used to measure the usability of telemedicine (Hajesmaeel-Gohari et al., 2021). Parmanto et al. (2016) developed the TUQ specifically to evaluate the usability of telemedicine and the implementation of the service, which impact the acceptance and adoption of the service by target end-users (Demiris et al., 2003, 2010).

Many aspects need to be considered when implementing telemedicine, including the feasibility, such as cost and resources available; technical capabilities; usability and acceptance by patients and physicians; clinical outcomes; and overall user satisfaction, among others. Thus, the TUQ can be an important instrument during a comprehensive and systematic telemedicine evaluation process.

The TUQ consists of 21 questions developed from existing telehealth questionnaires that comprehensively measure all aspects of usability (usefulness, ease of use and learnability, interface quality, interaction quality, reliability, satisfaction, and future use). The TUQ addresses the broad definition of usability to include an assessment of utility (whether the HIT's functionality does what users need) (Parmanto et al., 2016). The TUQ is able to be administered to both clinicians and patients, and can be used to assess various types of telehealth systems, such as traditional videoconferencing systems, computer-based systems, and newer mHealth platforms (Parmanto et al., 2016). Parmanto et al. (2016) assert that researchers should modify questions correctly to address various participants or telehealth systems.

Telemedicine Patient Questionnaire (TMPQ)

The Telemedicine Perception Questionnaire (TMPQ) is a 17-item survey that measures patients' acceptability of telemonitoring in terms of their perception of the risks and benefits (Demiris et al., 2000). The TMPQ is validated and free to use (Langbecker et al., 2017).

Telemedicine Satisfaction Questionnaire (TSQ)

Yip et al. (2003) developed the Telemedicine Satisfaction Questionnaire (TSQ) to evaluate patient satisfaction in using telemedicine (Hajesmaeel-Gohari et al., 2021). The TSQ consists of 14 items that assess parameters of the patient experience, such as difficulties in contacting therapist and willingness to use telemedicine (Yip et al., 2003).

Telemedicine Satisfaction and Usefulness Questionnaire (TSUQ)

Bakken (2006) developed both English and Spanish versions of the Telemedicine Satisfaction and Usefulness Questionnaire (TSUQ) to be able to evaluate urban and rural individuals' satisfaction and perception of usefulness of telemedicine. The TSUQ is a 26-item scale with 21 items focusing on perceived satisfaction with a five-point Likert scale rating of "strongly disagree" to "strongly agree" (Bakken, 2006). Five items focus on perceived usefulness with a five-point Likert scale rating ranging from "not at all useful" to "very useful" (Bakken, 2006). Results from the TSUQ allow researchers to explore relationships between telemedicine utilization in various geographic areas, and perceptions of satisfaction and usefulness.

Service User Technology Acceptability Questionnaire (SUTAQ)

Hirani et al. (2017) developed the Service User Technology Acceptability Questionnaire (SUTAQ) to judge users' acceptability of telemedicine services. The SUTAQ consists of 22 items that are categorized under six attributes:

benefits (nine items), privacy (four items), personal care skill (three items), substitution (three items), and satisfaction (three items) (Hirani et al., 2017). Hirani et al. (2017) suggest that the results of the SUTAQ discriminate between user groups and can be used to predict individual differences in beliefs and behaviors (Hirani et al., 2017).

ADDITIONAL-FOCUSED

After-Scenario Questionnaire (ASQ)

Lewis (1995) developed the After-Scenario Questionnaire (ASQ) as a simple three-item survey that is administered after each task or scenario in a usability test to measure how easy it was for participants to complete each task or scenario. Lewis (1995) asserts that it was important to assess user satisfaction during participation in a scenario-based usability test in addition measuring their perception of usability using the system after they have participated in a usability study as the PSSUQ measures. To this end, the ASQ instrument consists of three statements about which participants are asked to rate their level of agreement or disagreement according to a seven-point Likert scale with "1" equal to "strongly agree" and "7" equal to "strongly disagree." The three statements are:

1. Overall, I am satisfied with the ease of completing the task in this scenario.
2. Overall, I am satisfied with the amount of time it took to complete the task in this scenario.
3. Overall, I am satisfied with the support information (online help, messages, documentation) when completing the task.

According to this scale, *lower* scores indicate that participants felt the tasks were easy to perform and higher scores mean that participants found the tasks to be difficult or time-consuming. Similar to the Likert scale used in the PSSUQ, more recent studies use the reverse scale. The ASQ has acceptable psychometric properties of reliability, sensitivity, and concurrent validity (Lewis, 1991) and is a short, simple method for measuring perceived usability of a specific task or series of actions that users are likely to perform using a complex system.

AttrakDiff

The AttrakDiff is a validated pragmatic and hedonic metric of usability based on a semantic differential scale (Hassenzahl et al., 2003). The four qualities of usability the AttrakDiff measures include: pragmatic quality (PQ) related to effectiveness and efficiency, hedonic quality: identity (HQ-I) related to the self-image or self-expression of users as they use the product, hedonic quality: simulation (HQ-S) related to the perceived stimulation or excitement of the product when it is being used, and the general attractiveness (ATT) of the product (Takahashi & Nebe, 2019).

Client Satisfaction Questionnaire (CSQ)

The Client Satisfaction Questionnaire (CSQ) is a direct measure of consumer satisfaction with their service and is designed to be used with a wide range of client groups and service types, including health and human service (Attkisson & Zwick, 1982). The CSQ covers several aspects of service delivery and provision: physical surroundings; procedures; support staff; kind or type of service; treatment staff; quality of service; amount, length, or quantity of service; outcome of service; and general satisfaction (Attkisson et al., 1982).

End-User Computer Satisfaction (EUCS)

The End-User Computer Satisfaction (EUCS) was developed to measure end-user satisfaction of users who interact with a computer for a specific purpose by merging ease-of-use items and product information items (Doll & Torkzadeh, 1988). The EUCS consists of 12 items that cover five components of the user interaction: accuracy, content, format, timeliness, and ease of use (Doll et al., 1988).

NASA-Task Load Index (NASA-TLX)

The NASA-Task Load Index (NASA-TLX) is a survey that measures a user's mental workload (MWL) while performing a given task. The NASA-TLX rates performance across six dimensions and provides and overall workload rating: mental demand, physical demand, temporal demand, effort, performance, and frustration level (Stanton et al., 2017). The NASA-TLX is ideal for evaluating the mental effort required by a physician or patient to use a HIT successfully (Richardson et al., 2019).

Technology Acceptance Model (TAM)

The Technology Acceptance Model (TAM) aims to assess user acceptance of various technologies. Developed by Davis (1989), the TAM posits that users' acceptance and intention to use a technology is influenced by two primary factors: their perceived ease of use and perceived usefulness. There are two six-item scales that measure perceived ease of use and perceived usefulness that make-up the TAM. The original TAM asks respondents to rate their level of "likelihood" based on a seven-point Likert scale (Davis, 1989).

OTHER QUESTIONNAIRES AND SURVEYS

Given the sheer number of questionnaires and surveys that have been developed in the UX industry for various purposes, below I list others can be applied, given one's study, context, artifact under investigation, and type of insights about usability or UX one seeks to collect.

- Computer Usability Satisfaction Survey (CSUQ)
- Computer User Satisfaction Inventory (CUSI)
- Expectation Ratings (ER)
- Modular Evaluation of Components of User Experience (meCUE)
- Net Promotor Score (NPS)
- Purdue Usability Questionnaire (PUTQ)
- Service User Technology Acceptability Questionnaire (SUTAQ)
- Single Ease Question (SEQ)
- Software Usability Measurement Inventory (SUMI)
- Subject Mental Effort Question (SMEQ)
- System Causability Scale (SCS)
- UMUX-LITE
- Usability Magnitude Estimation (UME)
- User Experience Questionnaire (UEQ)
- Usefulness, Satisfaction, and Ease of use (USE) questionnaire

MODIFYING SCALES TO SUIT YOUR STUDY

Despite there being a plethora of psychometrically tested questionnaires and surveys that measure usability or some aspect of the UX, when there is no pre-existing data collection instrument that will enable you to garner the information you want to collect from end-users, develop one that will do this. Existing questionnaire and usability scales can be modified and added to in order to best apply to the artifact under investigation and collect insights on the aspects of usability or the UX you need. For instance, in the examination of the usability of telemedicine websites in a stationary context and mobile context, I developed the Telemedicine Interface Usability Questionnaire (TIUQ) as a retrospective questionnaire that was administered post-study to collect user insights into their UX (Campbell, 2020b). The TUIQ is a 12-item Likert scale that measures users' subjective perceptions of usability of telemedicine UIs (Campbell, 2020b). The TIUQ consists of 12 positive statements adapted from the SUS (Brooke, 1986), the PSSUQ (Lewis, 1992), and the TUQ (Parmanto et al., 2016) regarding the usability of the telemedicine provider interfaces, and asks subjects to respond with their level of agreement or disagreement on a five-point Likert scale with "1" meaning "I strongly disagree" and "5" meaning "I strongly agree" (Campbell, 2020b). Like the SUS, the TIUQ is a metric of users' overall impression of the usability of telemedicine interfaces with which they would interact in order to instigate a virtual physician visit, or virtual care.

WHAT SAMPLE SIZE DO I NEED?

Samples sizes for questionnaires and surveys vary depending on the target population and the reason for implanting a survey or questionnaire. If the research objective is to make inferences about a population or make comparisons in between or within subjects, then a larger sample population is recommended (Sauro & Lewis, personal communication, January 9, 2023; Sauro & Lewis, 2012). Of course, recruiting a sample population also depends on how narrow a population your study focuses on. For instance, the more screening criteria you have, the more difficult it will be for you to recruit a sizeable sample size. If you only require a general population, it will not be too difficult to recruit a large sample size. A good number to aim for is 100 participants for a survey or standardized questionnaire. If your survey or questionnaire is a post-study data collection instrument, then your sample population will be the same as that of your usability testing sample.

SUMMARY

This chapter presented several psychometrically tested, standardized surveys and questionnaires that quantitatively measure usability/UX or certain aspects of the UX. The system-agnostic SUS was discussed in detail, and many other HIT-specific questionnaires that measure usability were presented. Additionally, other aspects of the UX have well-known questionnaires aimed to capture that aspect, such as intention to use; these were also presented. The purpose of this chapter was to present the extensive questionnaires and surveys that quantitatively measure usability.

11

Conclusion

INTRODUCTION

This chapter concludes this book, and highlights some of key takeaways and messages that are important for readers to understand. It is understood that not every reader will need to or want to read every chapter and may navigate only to the chapters that are relevant to their study. Therefore, a brief chapter summary will be provided first, followed by an examination of the important messages that are infused into and reiterated throughout this book.

MIXED-METHODS EVALUATION OF HIT

Widespread adoption of health information technology (HIT), including EHRs, telemedicine, eHealth, and mHealth, necessitates that they be evaluated for usability to ensure they are safe and successfully implemented, and the outcomes are as expected—such as to improve health outcomes, as in the case of a digital health intervention (Zhang et al., 2019), or increase healthcare access, as in the case of telemedicine (Zhang et al., 2021).

Qualitative methods are generative and are able to collect data about UX that answer the "why?" questions regarding UX. Qualitative methods can be implemented in the formative and summative stages of the full system design lifecycle as they inform product design and capability decisions, as well as improving HIT usability through iterative refinements. Quantitative methods include field studies, interviews, and think-aloud usability testing. Findings from qualitative data offer an understanding of users' attitudes and motives for behaviors.

Quantitative methods are evaluative and involve measurements using numerical data. Findings from quantitative methods answer questions such as "how

DOI: 10.1201/9781003460886-11

many?" and "how much?" More often than not, quantitative methods are employed in the summative stages of the full system design lifecycle, and even after a HIT has been implemented, because the results are numerical and can be used as benchmarks for future usability testing. Some quantitative methods include eye tracking, analytics, and standardized scales, such as the SUS. Findings from quantitative methods offer evidence of users' behaviors.

Combined, the findings from qualitative and quantitative methods offer a more holistic understanding of UX. User-centered design (UCD) is a UX research and design process that involves users as participants early and often in the research and design process. UCD is often described as consisting of four stages that are iterative and focus on gaining a deep understanding of the target user of the HIT being developed to ensure the product meets the needs of the user and is usable and useful. It is important to note that the UCD process does not specify exact methods for each stage. It up to the researcher to determine which methods would best be implemented at any one stage during UCD. UCD involves the use of mixed-methods as you move through each of the stages of discovery, designing, prototyping, and testing. UCD is considered the most effective approach to designing usable products and is encouraged throughout this book.

The 2009 Health Information Technology for Economic and Clinical Health (HITECH) Act requires healthcare organizations to ensure "meaningful use" of HIT by certifying that HIT implemented has been usability tested (HITECH, 2009). As a part of the certification, the Office of the National Coordinator for Health Information Technology (ONC) requires vendors to provide evidence that UCD was employed along with the user testing results (HITECH, 2009; ONC, 2012). Therefore, the impetus to design and develop usable HIT by employing UCD is strong.

SUMMARY

This book was written for a wide audience of health information UX researchers, designers, and providers, together with healthcare professionals and technical communicators to be able to conduct quality UX research and inform the design of usable HIT. This book was also written for scholars, academics, instructors, and graduate students to use as a reference manual, course textbook, and research tool, as it is filled with practical and tactic knowledge regarding usability engineering and UCD applied in the healthcare sector.

- *Chapter 1: Introduction.* This introductory chapter broadly defined HIT and the impetus for performing mixed-methods usability studies of HIT. It also provided an overview of the information presented in the book and how the book was organized. It provided evidence for the exigency of usable HIT in today's modern, digitalized society.

- *Chapter 2: Definitions: Usability, UX, and UCD.* This chapter offered many definitions of usability that have been developed and used in the fields of technical communication, HCI, and UX. Usefulness was discussed as an independent variable, but is required for HIT adoption by users. The implications of usability on the user experience were also discussed. Lastly, the user-centered design (UCD) process was described as an iterative design lifecycle that includes all stakeholders (clinicians, patients, researchers, etc.). It briefly introduced the subsequent chapters on individual and contextual determinants of usability and the various usability testing methods used in the formative and summative stages of the UCD/full system design lifecycle.

- *Chapter 3: Audience Analysis and Usability Determinants.* This chapter discussed the multidimensional factors affecting usability by distinguishing individual/subjective and contextual/external factors: cognitive, social, physical, environmental, etc. It explained formative and summative usability testing and the methods used for each type, as well as examining the stage of the UCD process in which each testing method occurs.

- *Chapter 4: Quantitative and Qualitative Methods.* This chapter defined and explained quantitative and qualitative methods, and looked at the types of data obtained from using each method, how the data are analyzed, and what can be concluded or inferred from each method.

- *Chapter 5: Mixed-methods Study Design and Rigor.* This chapter asserted that mixed-methods are a beneficial approach to conducing comprehensive and valuable usability studies of health information technology. It aimed to inform researchers on how to approach the design of a mixed-methods study by first identifying their object of inquiry (the technology being studied) and what they want to discover about usability (development of their research questions), so they can select the best methods, as explained in subsequent chapters. The chapter discussed the affordances (rich data corpus, greater interaction with data, more usability metrics can be measured) and limitations (resource-intensive, costly, timely) of employing mixed-methods. Lastly, it addressed how scientific studies are considered rigorous and how the quality of one's study is evaluated differently depending on whether the study is quantitative or qualitative. The

criteria for evaluating the rigor of a study were defined, including generalizability, validity, and fidelity. An explanation of data triangulation and
feasibility was also included.

- *Chapter 6: Content Analysis.* This chapter described the research methodology and content analysis, and offered various coding techniques and
ways of approaching how to make sense of a wide variety of qualitative
data, including using a framework approach, inductive coding, and an a
priori coding scheme. Content analysis is a method to discover what type
of health communications exist, which helps explicate the problem with
existing technology, lack of usable technology, or lack of understanding
what the user needs to be able to do with the technology. The coding
techniques introduced in this chapter can be applied to analyze data
collected from usability testing methods described in subsequent chapters,
such as cognitive walkthroughs and think-alouds.

- *Chapter 7: Discovery UX Research Studies.* This chapter described the types
of inquiry that should be used prior to beginning to design a HIT product.
It focused on formative testing, where the researcher is conducting user
research and seeking to discover how target users will actually interact
with the product they are designing and what contextual and subjective
factors affect usability. The methods discussed in this chapter are focused
on understanding the users for whom the HIT is being designed, what
they intend to use it for, the types of interactions they may have with the
product, and the context in which the HIT will be used. Both formal
and informal methods were discussed, including field observations, diary
studies, focus groups, interviews, and surveys.

- *Chapter 8: Usability Inspection Methods.* This chapter described more traditional formative usability testing methods, such as those conducted with
experts only and those with end-users. It explained how to perform the
various usability testing techniques that generally obtain qualitative data,
such as think-aloud usability testing, including how many representative users are needed, how to recruit human subjects, developing real-life
testing scenarios, and in what context to perform the study.

- *Chapter 9: Quantitative Usability Testing Methods and Metrics.* This
chapter described how to perform various usability tests that generally
obtain quantitative data and how this data can be attributed to usability
problems, such as frequency of task completion success versus failure and
eye-tracking data. It covered summative methods that can be completed
after a HIT has been implemented and is already being used.

- *Chapter 10: Post-study Surveys and Retrospective Questionnaires.* This chapter introduced several standardized scales that measure UX or some aspect of UX, including the post popular and highly leveraged System Usability Scale (SUS). Several other common post-study usability scales were introduced, including the Post-study System Usability Questionnaire (PSSUQ), the Telemedicine Satisfaction and Usefulness Questionnaire (TSUQ), the Questionnaire for User Interface Satisfaction (QUIS), and the NASA-Task Load Index (NASA-TLX).
- *Chapter 11: Conclusion.* This concluding chapter has summarized the key takeaways of the text: develop research inquiries and select the best mixture of methods that will allow you to answer your research questions. It has encouraged readers to perform interdisciplinary, collaborative research and mix methods, and to use the information to iteratively design usable HIT.

FINAL THOUGHTS

Finally, while UCD requires a collaborative approach with users, it would be best informed by interdisciplinary knowledge. The variety of methods that can be employed in mixed-methods studies, in addition to the numerous approaches and techniques for analyzing data, makes it difficult to be an expert in every single method. Therefore, it is best to engage with an interdisciplinary team of people who can offer knowledge from a variety of disciplines and experiences. Interdisciplinary collaboration affords multiple perspectives and ways to approach a problem, and expands a single researcher's ability to explore a phenomenon and develop solutions. Collaboration inspires innovation.

References

Abdulrahman Mohammed Al, M., Zakiuddin, A., & Abdullah M., A. (2018). Paradigm shift in healthcare through technology and patient-centeredness. *International Archives of Public Health and Community Medicine*, 2(1). https://doi.org/10.23937/iaphcm-2017/1710015

Ackerman, S., Gleason, N., & Gonzales, R. (2015). Using rapid ethnography to support the design and implementation of health information technologies. *Techno-Anthropology in Health Informatics*, 215, 14–27. https://doi.org/10.3233/978-1-61499-560-9-14

Agarwal, R., Anderson, C., Zarate, J., & Ward, C. (2013). If we offer it, will they accept? Factors affecting patient use intentions of personal health records and secure messaging. *Journal of Medical Internet research*, 15(2), e43. https://doi.org/10.2196/jmir.2243

Agha, Z., Schapira, R. M., Laud, P. W., McNutt, G., & Roter, D. L. (2009). Patient satisfaction with physician–patient communication during telemedicine. *Telemedicine Journal and e-Health: The Official Journal of the American Telemedicine Association*, 15(9), 830–839. https://doi.org/10.1089/tmj.2009.0030

Agnisarman, S. O., Madathil, K. C., Smith, K., Ashoka, A., Welch, B., & McElligott, J. T. (2017). Lessons learned from the usability assessment of home-based telemedicine systems. *Applied Ergonomics*, 58, 424–434.

Agree, E. M., King, A. C., Castro, C. M., Wiley, A., & Borzekowski, D. L. (2015). "It's got to be on this page": Age and cognitive style in a study of online health information seeking. *Journal of Medical Internet Research*, 17(3), e79. https://doi.org/10.2196/jmir.3352

Ahmad, S., Wasim, S., Irfan, S., Gogoi, S., Srivastava, A., & Farheen, Z. (2019). Qualitative vs. quantitative research: A summarized review. *Journal of Evidence Based Medicine and Healthcare*, 6, 2828–2832.

Aitken L. M., Marshall, A., Elliott, R., & McKinley, S. (2011). Comparison of "think aloud" and observation as data collection methods in the study of decision making regarding sedation in intensive care patients. *International Journal of Nursing Studies*, 48(3), 318–325. https://doi.org/101016/j.ijnurstu.2010.07.014

Alaiad, A., & Zhou, L. (2017). Patients' adoption of WSN-based smart home healthcare systems: An integrated model of facilitators and barriers. *IEEE Transactions on Professional Communication*, 60(1), 4–23. https://doi.org/10.1109/TPC.2016.2632822

Alami, J., Hammonds, C., Hensien, E., Khraibani, J., Borowitz, S., Hellems, M., & Riggs, S. L. (2022). Usability challenges with electronic health records (EHRs) during prerounding on pediatric inpatients. *JAMIA Open*, 5(1), 18. https://doi.org/10.1093/jamiaopen/ooac018

Alathas, H. (2018, November 19). How to measure product usability with the System Usability Scale (SUS) score. *UX Planet*. Retrieved from https://uxplanet.org/how-to-measure-product-usability-with-the-system-usability-scale-sus-score-69f3875b858f

Albers, M. J. (2003). Multidimensional audience analysis for dynamic information. *Journal of Technical Writing and Communication*, 33(3), 263–279. https://doi.org/10.2190/6KJN-95QV-JMD3-E5EE

Alotaibi, Y. K., & Federico, F. (2017). The impact of health information technology on patient safety. *Saudi Medical Journal*, 38(12), 1173–1180. https://doi.org/10.15537/smj.2017.12.20631

Alpert, J. M., Krist, A. H., Aycock, R. A., & Kreps, G. L. (2017). Designing user-centric patient portals: Clinician and patients' uses and gratifications. *Telemedicine Journal and E-Health*, 23(3), 248–253. https://doi.org/10.1089/tmj.2016.0096

Alroobaea, R., & Mayhew, P. J. (2014). How many participants are really enough for usability studies? In *Proceedings of 2014 Science and Information Conference, SAI 2014*. The Institute of Electrical and Electronics Engineers (IEEE), 48–56. https://doi.org/10.1109/SAI.2014.6918171

Alrubaiee, L. (2011). The mediating effect of patient satisfaction in the patients' perceptions of healthcare quality: Patient trust relationship. *International Journal of Marketing Studies*, 3(1), 103–127.

Alzougool, B., Chang, S., & Gray, K. (2008). Towards a comprehensive understanding of health information needs. *Electronic Journal of Health Informatics*, 3(2): e15. Retrieved from www.academia.edu/16967764

Ammenwerth, E. (2015). Evidence-based health informatics: How do we know what we know? *Methods of Information in Medicine*, 54(4), 298–307. https://doi.org/10.3414/ME14-01-0119

Aristotle. (1991). *On rhetoric: A theory of civic discourse*. (G. A. Kennedy, Trans.). Oxford University Press. (Original work published ca. 350 BCE)

Artnak, K. E., McGraw, R. M., & Stanley, V. F. (2011). Health care accessibility for chronic illness management and end-of-life care: A view from rural America. *Journal of Law, Medicine & Ethics*, 39(2), 140–155. https://doi.org/10.1111/j.1748-720X.2011.00584.x

Asan, O., & Yang, Y. (2015). Using eye trackers for usability evaluation of health information technology: A systematic literature review. *JMIR Human Factors*, 2(1), e5. https://doi.org/10.2196/humanfactors.4062

ATLAS.ti. (n.d.). *The qualitative data analysis & research software*. Retrieved from https://atlasti.com

Attkisson, C. C., & Zwick, R. (1982). The client satisfaction questionnaire. *Evaluation and Program Planning*, 5(3), 233–237. https://doi.org/10.1016/0149-7189(82)90074-X

Bailey, C., White, C., & Pain, R. (1999). Evaluating qualitative research: Dealing with the tension between "science" and "creativity." *Area*, 31(2), 169–178. Retrieved from www.jstor.org/stable/20003972

Bakken, S., Grullon-Figueroa, L., Izquierdo, R., Lee, N.-J., Morin, P., Palmas, W., Teresi, J., Weinstock, R. S., Shea, S., Starren, J., & IDEATel Consortium. (2006). Development, validation, and use of English and Spanish versions of the Telemedicine Satisfaction and Usefulness Questionnaire. *Journal of the American Medical Informatics Association*, 13(6), 660–667. https://doi.org/10.1197/jamia.M2146

Bandura, A. (1982). Self-efficacy mechanism in human agency. *American Psychologist*, 37(2), 122–147.

Bangor, A., Kortum, P., & Miller, J. (2009). Determining what individual SUS scores mean: Adding an adjective rating scale. *Journal of Usability Studies*, 4(3). 114–213.

Bashshur, R. L. (1995). On the definition and evaluation of telemedicine. *Telemedicine Journal: The Official Journal of the American Telemedicine Association*, 1(1), 19–30. https://doi.org/10.1089/tmj.1.1995.1.19

Beck, K. (2000). *Extreme programming explained: Embrace change*. Addison-Wesley.

Bengtsson, M. (2016). How to plan and perform a qualitative study using content analysis. *NursingPlus Open*, 2, 8–14. https://doi.org/10.1016/j.npls.2016.01.001

Berg, B. L., Lune, H., & Lune, H. (2004). *Qualitative research methods for the social sciences*. Pearson.

Berkman, N. D., Sheridan, S. L., Donahue, K. E., Halpern, D. J., & Crotty, K. (2011). Low health literacy and health outcomes: An updated systematic review. *Annals of Internal Medicine*, 155(2), 97–107. https://doi.org/10.7326/0003-4819-155-2-201107190-00005

Beyer, H., & Holtzblatt, K. (1998). *Contextual design: Defining customer-centered systems*. Morgan Kaufmann.

Bhutkar, G., Konkani, A., Katre, D., & Ray, G. G. (2013). A review: Healthcare usability evaluation methods. *Biomedical Instrumentation & Technology*, 47(s2), 45–53. https://doi.org/10.2345/0899-8205-47.s2.45

Billson, J. (1989). Focus groups: A practical guide for applied research. *Clinical Sociology Review*, 7(1). Retrieved from https://digitalcommons.wayne.edu/csr/vol7/iss1/24

Birru, M. S., Monaco, V. M., Charles, L., Drew, H., Njie, V., Bierria, T., ... Steinman R. A. (2004). Internet usage by low-literacy adults seeking health information: An observational analysis. *Journal of Medical Internet Research*, 6(3), e25. https://doi.org/10.2196/jmir.6.3.e25

Blödt, S., Pach, D., Roll, S., & Witt, C. M. (2014). Effectiveness of app-based relaxation for patients with chronic low back pain (Relaxback) and chronic neck pain (Relaxneck): Study protocol for two randomized pragmatic trials. *Trials*, 15(1), 490. https://doi.org/10.1186/1745-6215-15-490

Bodie, G. D., & Dutta, M. J. (2008). Understanding health literacy for strategic health marketing: eHealth literacy, health disparities, and the digital divide. *Health Marketing Quarterly*, 25(1–2), 175–203. https://doi.org/10.1080/07359680802126301

Boettger, R. K., & Palmer, L. A. (2010). Quantitative content analysis: Its use in technical communication. *IEEE Transactions on Professional Communication*, 53(4), 346–357. https://doi.org/10.1109/TPC.2010.2077450

Bolger, N., Davis, A., & Rafaeli, E. (2003). Diary methods: Capturing life as it is Lived. *Annual Review of Psychology*, 54(1), 579–616. https://doi.org/10.1146/annurev.psych.54.101601.145030

Bollmeier, S. G., Stevenson, E., Finnegan, P., & Griggs, S. K. (2020). Direct to consumer telemedicine: Is healthcare from home best? *Missouri Medicine*, 117(4), 303–309.

Borycki, E. (Ed.). (2011). *International perspectives in health informatics*. IOS Press.

Borycki, E. M., & Kushniruk, A. W. (2010). Towards an integrative cognitive-socio-technical approach in health informatics: Analyzing technology-induced error involving health information systems to improve patient safety. *The Open Medical Informatics Journal*, 4, 181–187. https://doi.org/10.2174/1874431101004010181

Borycki, E. M., Kushniruk, A. W., Kuwata, S., & Kannry, J. (2011). Engineering the electronic health record for safety: A multi-level video-based approach to diagnosing and preventing technology-induced error arising from usability problems. *Studies in Health Technology and Informatics*, 166, 197–205.

Borycki, E., & Kushniruk, A. (2005). Identifying and preventing technology-induced error using simulations: Application of usability engineering techniques. *Healthcare Quarterly*, 8, 99–105. https://doi.org/10.12927/hcq..17673

Borycki, E., Kushniruk, A., Nohr, C., Takeda, H., Kuwata, S., Carvalho, C., Bainbridge, M., & Kannry, J. (2013). Usability methods for ensuring health information technology safety: Evidence-based approaches. Contribution of the IMIA working group health informatics for patient safety. *Yearbook of Medical Informatics*, 8, 20–27.

Bradway, M., Giordanengo, A., Joakimsen, R., Hansen, A. H., Grøttland, A., Hartvigsen, G., Randine, P., & Årsand, E. (2020). Measuring the effects of sharing mobile health data during diabetes consultations: Protocol for a mixed method study. *JMIR Research Protocols*, 9(2), e16657. https://doi.org/10.2196/16657

Bright, T. J., Bakken, S., & Johnson, S. B. (2006). Heuristic evaluation of eNote: An electronic notes system. *AMIA Annual Symposium Proceedings*, 864. Retrieved from www.ncbi.nlm. nih.gov/pmc/articles/PMC1839434

Broekhuis, M., van Velsen, L., & Hermens, H. (2019). Assessing usability of eHealth technology: A comparison of usability benchmarking instruments. *International Journal of Medical Informatics*, 128, 24–31. https://doi.org/10.1016/j.ijmedinf.2019.05.001

Brooke, J. (1986). *SUS: A quick and dirty usability scale*. Reading, United Kingdom: Digital Equipment Corporation.

Brooke, J. (2013). SUS: A retrospective. *Journal of Usability Studies*, 8(2), 29–40.

Brown, W., Yen, P.-Y., Rojas, M., & Schnall, R. (2013). Assessment of the Health IT Usability Evaluation Model (Health-ITUEM) for evaluating mobile health (mHealth) technology. *Journal of Biomedical Informatics*, 46(6), 1080–1087. https://doi.org/10.1016/j.jbi.2013.08.001

Brunner, J., Chuang, E., Goldzweig, C., Cain, C. L., Sugar, C., & Yano, E. M. (2017). User-centered design to improve clinical decision support in primary care. *International Journal of Medical Informatics*, 104, 56–64. https://doi.org/10.1016/j.ijmedinf.2017.05.004

Bruno, V., & al-Qaimari, G. (2004). Usability attributes: An initial step toward effective user-centred development. In *Proceedings of OZHI2004*. Retrieved from http://citeseerx.ist.psu.edu/viewdoc/summary?doi=10.1.1.83.662

Bryant, M. J., Ward, D. S., Hales, D., Vaughn, A., Tabak, R. G., & Stevens, J. (2008). Reliability and validity of the Healthy Home Survey: A tool to measure factors within homes hypothesized to relate to overweight in children. *International Journal of Behavioral Nutrition and Physical Activity*, 5(1), 23. https://doi.org/10.1186/1479-5868-5-23

Buchanan, C., Threatt, A., Weinger, M., & Miller, A. (2014). High variability in summative usability test methods & reporting among clinical informatics vendors complying with Federal certification requirements. *Proceedings of the Human Factors and Ergonomics Society Annual Meeting*, 58, 1491–1495. https://doi.org/10.1177/1541931214581311

Buchanan, S., & Salako, A. (2009). Evaluating the usability and usefulness of a digital library. *Library Review*, 58(9), 638–651. https://doi.org/10.1108/00242530910997928

Budiu, R. (2021, June 27). Confidence intervals, margins of error, and confidence levels in UX. Nielsen Norman Group. Retrieved from www.nngroup.com/articles/confidence-interval

Campbell, J. L. (2020a). A mixed-methods approach to evaluating the usability of telemedicine communications. *Proceedings of the 38th ACM International Conference on Design of Communication*, 1–6. https://doi.org/10.1145/3380851.3416755

Campbell, J. L. (2020b). *Examining the design and usability of telemedicine communications: A mixed-methods study*. Doctoral dissertation, University of Central Florida. Retrieved from https://stars.library.ucf.edu/etd2020/189; https://purls.library.ucf.edu/go/DP0023475

Campbell, J. L. (2020c). Healthcare experience design: A conceptual and methodological framework for understanding the effects of usability on the access, delivery, and receipt of healthcare. *Knowledge Management & e-Learning*, 12(4), 505–520. https://doi.org/10.34105/j.kmel.2020.12.028

Campbell, J. L. (2023). Identifying digital rhetoric in the telemedicine user interface. *Journal of Technical Writing and Communication*, 53(2), 89–105. https://doi.org/10.1177/004728 16221125184

Campbell, J. L., & Monkman, H. (2021). The application of a novel, context specific, remote, usability assessment tool to conduct a pre-redesign and post-redesign usability comparison of a telemedicine website. *Studies in Health Technology and Informatics*, 281, 911–915. https://doi.org/10.3233/SHTI210311

Campbell, J. L., & Monkman, H. (2022). Pre- and post-redesign usability assessment of a telemedicine interface based on subjective metrics. *Studies in Health Technology and Informatics*, 290, 872–876. https://doi.org/10.3233/SHTI220204

Card, S. K., Moran, T. P., & Newell, A. (1980). The keystroke-level model for user performance time with interactive systems. *Communications of the ACM*, 23, 396–410.

Card, S., Moran, T., & Newell, A. (1983). *The psychology of human–computer interaction*. Lawrence Erlbaum.

Carliner, S. (2000). Physical, cognitive, and affective: A three-part framework for information design. *Technical Communication*, 47(4), 561–576.

Carroll, J. M. (1997). Human–computer interaction: Psychology as a science of design. *International Journal of Human-Computer Studies*, 46(4), 501–522. https://doi.org/10.1006/ijhc.1996.0101

Carroll, J. M., & Campbell, R. L. (1987). Softening up hard science: Reply to Newell and Card. In P. Zunde & J. C. Agrawal (Eds.), *Empirical foundations of information and software science* (pp. 13–31). Springer. https://doi.org/10.1007/978-1-4684-5472-7_5

Carroll, J. M., & McKendree, J. (1986). Interface design issues for advice-giving expert systems. *Communications of the ACM*, 30(1), 14–31.

Cartwright, D. (1953). Analysis of qualitative material. In L. Festinger & D. Katz (Eds.), *Research methods in the behavioral sciences* (pp. 421–470). Dryden Press.

Carvalho, C., Borycki, E., & Kushniruk, A. (2009). Ensuring the safety of health information systems: Using heuristics for patient safety. *Healthcare Quarterly*, 12, 49–54. https://doi.org/10.12927/hcq.2009.20966

Cavanagh, S. (1997). Content analysis: Concepts, methods and applications. *Nurse Researcher*, 4(3), 5–16. https://doi.org/10.7748/nr.4.3.5.s2

Champlin, S., Cuculick, J., Hauser, P. C., Wyse, K., & McKee, M. M. (2021). Using gaze tracking as a research tool in the Deaf Health Literacy and Access to Health Information Project: Protocol for a multisite mixed methods study and preliminary results. *JMIR Research Protocols*, 10(9), e26708. https://doi.org/10.2196/26708

Chen, A. T., Wu, S., Tomasino, K. N., Lattie, E. G., & Mohr, D. C. (2019). A multi-faceted approach to characterizing user behavior and experience in a digital mental health intervention. *Journal of Biomedical Informatics*, 94, 103187. https://doi.org/10.1016/j.jbi.2019.103187

Chew, C., & Eysenbach, G. (2010). Pandemics in the age of Twitter: Content analysis of tweets during the 2009 H1N1 outbreak. *PLoS ONE*, 5(11), e14118. https://doi.org/10.1371/journal.pone.0014118

Chin, J. P., Diehl, V. A., & Norman, L. K. (1988). Development of an instrument measuring user satisfaction of the human–computer interface. *Proceedings of the SIGCHI Conference on Human Factors in Computing Systems—CHI '88*, 213–218. https://doi.org/10.1145/57167.57203

Cho, H., Keenan, G., Madandola, O. O., Santos, F. C. D., Macieira, T. G. R., Bjarnadottir, R. I., Priola, K. J. B., & Lopez, K. D. (2022). Assessing the usability of a clinical decision support system: Heuristic evaluation. *JMIR Human Factors*, 9(2), e31758. https://doi.org/10.2196/31758

Cho, J., & Lee, E.-H. (2014). Reducing confusion about grounded theory and qualitative content analysis: Similarities and differences. *The Qualitative Report*, 19(64). https://doi.org/10.46743/2160-3715/2014.1028

Choi, N. G., Wilson, N. L., Sirrianni, L., Marinucci, M. L., & Hegel, M. T. (2014). Acceptance of home-based telehealth problem-solving therapy for depressed, low-income homebound older adults: Qualitative interviews with the participants and aging-service case managers. *The Gerontologist*, 54, 704–713. https://doi.org/10.1093/geront/gnt083

Choudhury, A., Elkefi, S., Strachna, O., & Asan, O. (2022). Effect of patient portals on perception of care quality, general health, and mental health: An exploratory analysis. *Human Factors in Healthcare*, 2, 100018. https://doi.org/10.1016/j.hfh.2022.100018

Ciere, Y., Jaarsma, D., Visser, A., Sanderman, R., Snippe, E., & Fleer, J. (2015). Studying learning in the healthcare setting: The potential of quantitative diary methods. *Perspectives on Medical Education*, 4(4), 203–207. https://doi.org/10.1007/s40037-015-0199-3

Cline, R., & Haynes, K. (2001). Consumer health information seeking on the internet: The state of the art. *Health Education Research*, 16, 671–692.

Cohen, J. (1988). *Statistical power analysis for the behavioral sciences* (2nd ed). Lawrence Erlbaum.

Creswell, J. W. (2002). *Educational research: Planning, conducting, and evaluating quantitative and qualitative research* (4th ed.). Pearson.

Cronbach, L. J., & Meehl, P. E. (1955). Construct validity for psychological tests. *Psychological Bulletin*, 52, 281–302. Retrieved from http://psychclassics.yorku.ca/Cronbach/construct.htm#f1

Cropley, A. J. (2019). *Qualitative research methods: A practice-oriented introduction for students of psychology and education.* (2nd ed.). Zinātne.

Curry, L. A., Nembhard, I. M., & Bradley, E. H. (2009). Qualitative and mixed methods provide unique contributions to outcomes research. *Circulation*, 119(10), 1442–1452. https://doi.org/10.1161/CIRCULATIONAHA.107.742775

Cypress, B. S. (2017). Rigor or reliability and validity in qualitative research: Perspectives, strategies, reconceptualization, and recommendations. *Dimensions of Critical Care Nursing*, 36(4), 253–263. https://doi.org/10.1097/DCC.0000000000000253

Damman, O. C., Hendriks, M., Rademakers, J., Delnoij, D. M., & Groenewegen, P. P. (2009). How do healthcare consumers process and evaluate comparative healthcare information? A qualitative study using cognitive interviews. *BMC Public Health*, 9(1), 423. https://doi.org/10.1186/1471-2458-9-423

Dang, S., Remon, N., Harris, J., Malphurs, J., Sandals, L., Cabrera, A. L., & Nedd, N. (2008). Care coordination assisted by technology for multiethnic caregivers of persons with dementia: A pilot clinical demonstration project on caregiver burden and depression. *Journal of Telemedicine & Telecare*, 14(8), 443–447. https://doi.org/10.1258/jtt.2008.080608

Daniëls, N. E. M., Hochstenbach, L. M. J., van Zelst, C., van Bokhoven, M. A., Delespaul, P. A. E. G., & Beurskens, A. J. H. M. (2021). Factors that influence the use of electronic diaries in health care: Scoping review. *JMIR MHealth and UHealth*, 9(6), e19536. https://doi.org/10.2196/19536

Davis, F. (1989). Perceived usefulness, perceived ease of use, and user acceptance of information technology. *MIS Quarterly*, 13(3), 319–340. https://doi.org/10.2307/249008

de Souza, C. H. A., Morbeck, R. A., Steinman, M., Hors, C. P., Bracco, M. M., Kozasa, E. H., & Leão, E. R. (2017). Barriers and benefits in telemedicine arising between a high-technology hospital service provider and remote public healthcare units: A qualitative study in Brazil. *Telemedicine and e-Health*, 23(6), 527–532. https://doi.org/10.1089/tmj.2016.0158

Delmar, C. (2010). "Generalizability" as recognition: Reflections on a foundational problem in qualitative research. *Qualitative Studies*, 1, 115–128.

Demiris, G., Charness, N., Krupinski, E., Ben-Arieh, D., Washington, K., Wu, C.-H., & Bonne, F. (2010). The role of human factors in telehealth. *Telemedicine Journal and e-Health: The*

Official Journal of the American Telemedicine Association, 16, 446–453. https://doi.org/10.1089/tmj.2009.0114

Demiris, G., Speedie, S., & Finkelstein, S. (2000). A questionnaire for the assessment of patients' impressions of the risks and benefits of home telecare. *Journal of Telemedicine and Telecare*, 6(5), 278–284. https://doi.org/10.1258/1357633001935914

Demiris, G., Speedie, S., Finkelstein, S., & Harris, I. (2003). Communication patterns and technical quality of virtual visits in home care. *Journal of Telemedicine and Telecare*, 9(4), 210–215.

Devine, E. B., Hansen, R. N., Wilson-Norton, J. L., Lawless, N. M., Fisk, A. W., Blough, D. K., Martin, D. P., & Sullivan, S. D. (2010). The impact of computerized provider order entry on medication errors in a multispecialty group practice. *Journal of the American Medical Informatics Association*, 17(1), 78–84. https://doi.org/10.1197/jamia.M3285

Dewalt, D. A., Berkman, N. D., Sheridan, S., Lohr, K. N., & Pignone, M. P. (2004). Literacy and health outcomes: a systematic review of the literature. *Journal of General Internal Medicine*, 19(12), 1228–1239. https://doi.org/10.1111/j.1525-1497.2004.40153.x

Diaper, D., & Stanton, N. A. (Eds.). (2004). *The handbook of task analysis for human–computer interaction*. Lawrence Erlbaum.

Dicicco-Bloom, B., & Crabtree, B. F. (2006). The qualitative research interview. *Medical Education*, 40(4), 314–321. https://doi.org/10.1111/j.1365-2929.2006.02418.x

Dix, A., Finlay, J., Abowd, G. D., & Beale, R. (Eds.). (2004). *Human–computer interaction* (3rd ed.). Pearson Prentice-Hall.

Djamasbi, S., Tullis, T., Hsu, J., Mazuera, E., Osberg, K., & Bosch, J. (2007). Gender preferences in web design: Usability testing through eye tracking. *AMCIS 2007 Proceedings*. Retrieved from https://aisel.aisnet.org/amcis2007/133

Doberne, J. W., He, Z., Mohan, V., Gold, J. A., Marquard, J., & Chiang, M. F. (2015). Using high-fidelity simulation and eye tracking to characterize EHR workflow patterns among hospital physicians. *AMIA Annual Symposium Proceedings*, 1881–1889.

Doll, W. J., & Torkzadeh, G. (1988). The measurement of end-user computing satisfaction. *MIS Quarterly*, 12(2), 259–274. https://doi.org/10.2307/248851

Doran, D. M., Mylopoulos, J., Kushniruk, A., Nagle, L., Laurie-Shaw, B., Sidani, S., Tourangeau, A. E., Lefebre, N., Reid-Haughian, C., Carryer, J. R., Cranley, L. A., & McArthur, G. (2007). Evidence in the palm of your hand: Development of an outcomes-focused knowledge translation intervention. *Worldviews on Evidence-Based Nursing*, 4(2), 69–77. https://doi.org/10.1111/j.1741-6787.2007.00084.x

Dovetail. (n.d.). Dovetail Research Pty Ltd website. Retrieved from https://dovetail.com

Dowding, D., Merrill, J. A., Barrón, Y., Onorato, N., Jonas, K., & Russell, D. (2019). Usability evaluation of a dashboard for home care nurses. *CIN: Computers, Informatics, Nursing*, 37(1), 11. https://doi.org/10.1097/CIN.0000000000000484

dscout. (2023). dscout for healthcare. Retrieved from https://dscout.com/industries/healthcare

Dumas, J. S., & Redish, J. (1999). *A practical guide to usability testing*. Intellect.

Duncan, B. J., Kaufman, D. R., Zheng, L., Grando, A., Furniss, S. K., Poterack, K. A., Miksch, T. A., Helmers, R. A., & Doebbeling, B. N. (2020). A micro-analytic approach to understanding electronic health record navigation paths. *Journal of Biomedical Informatics*, 110, 103566. https://doi.org/10.1016/j.jbi.2020.103566

Dutta-Bergman, M. (2003). Trusted online sources of health information: differences in demographics, health beliefs, and health-information orientation. *Journal of medical internet research*, 5(3), e21. Retrieved from www.ncbi.nlm.nih.gov/pmc/articles/PMC1550562/

Dutta-Bergman, M. (2004). Primary sources of health information: Comparisons in the domain of health attitudes, health cognitions, and health behaviors. *Health Communication, 16*(3), 273–288.

Egan, D. E. (1988). Individual differences in human-computer interaction. In M. Helander (Ed.), *Handbook of human–computer interaction* (pp. 543–568). Elsevier.

Eghdam, A., Forsman, J., Falkenhav, M., Lind, M., & Koch, S. (2011). Combining usability testing with eye-tracking technology: Evaluation of a visualization support for antibiotic use in intensive care. *Studies in Health Technology and Informatics, 169*, 945–949.

Elo, S., Kääriäinen, M., Kanste, O., Pölkki, T., Utriainen, K., & Kyngäs, H. (2014). Qualitative content analysis: A focus on trustworthiness. *SAGE Open, 4*(1), 2158244014522633. https://doi.org/10.1177/2158244014522633

Ericsson, K. A., & Simon, H. A. (1980). Verbal reports as data. *Psychological Review, 87*(3), 215–251.

Ericsson, K. A., & Simon, H. (1984). *Protocol analysis: Verbal reports as data.* MIT Press.

Erlandson, D. A. (Ed.). (1993). *Doing naturalistic inquiry: A guide to methods.* Sage.

Erlingsson, C., & Brysiewicz, P. (2017). A hands-on guide to doing content analysis. *African Journal of Emergency Medicine, 7*(3), 93–99. https://doi.org/10.1016/j.afjem.2017.08.001

Erol Barkana, D., & Açık, A. (2014). Improvement of design of a surgical interface using an eye tracking device. *Theoretical Biology and Medical Modelling, 11*(S1), S4. https://doi.org/10.1186/1742-4682-11-S1-S4

Eysenbach, G. (2000). Consumer health informatics. *British Medical Journal, 320*(7251), 1713–1716.

Eysenbach, G. (2005). Design and evaluation of consumer health information web sites. In D. Lewis, G. Eysenbach, R. Kukafka, P. Z. Stavri, & H. B. Jimison (Eds.), *Consumer health informatics: Informing consumers and improving health care* (pp. 34–60). Springer. https://doi.org/10.1007/0-387-27652-1_4

Eysenbach, G., & Köhler, C. (2002). How do consumers search for and appraise health information on the world wide web? Qualitative study using focus groups, usability tests, and in-depth interviews. *British Medical Journal, 324*, 573–577.

Fabricius, P. K., Andersen, O., Steffensen, K. D., & Kirk, J. W. (2021). The challenge of involving old patients with polypharmacy in their medication during hospitalization in a medical emergency department: An ethnographic study. *PLoS ONE, 16*(12), e0261525. https://doi.org/10.1371/journal.pone.0261525

Farrahi, R., Rangraz Jeddi, F., Nabovati, E., Sadeqi Jabali, M., & Khajouei, R. (2019). The relationship between user interface problems of an admission, discharge and transfer module and usability features: A usability testing method. *BMC Medical Informatics and Decision Making, 19*(1), 172. https://doi.org/10.1186/s12911-019-0893-x

Farzandipour, M., Nabovati, E., & Sadeqi Jabali, M. (2022). Comparison of usability evaluation methods for a health information system: Heuristic evaluation versus cognitive walk-through method. *BMC Medical Informatics and Decision Making, 22*(1), 157. https://doi.org/10.1186/s12911-022-01905-7

Faulkner, L. (2003). Beyond the five-user assumption: Benefits of increased sample sizes in usability testing. *Behavior Research Methods, Instruments, & Computers, 35*(3), 379–383. https://doi.org/10.3758/BF03195514

Finstad, K. (2010). The usability metric for user experience. *Interacting with Computers, 22*(5), 323–327. https://doi.org/10.1016/j.intcom.2010.04.004

Fontana, A., & Frey, J. H. (2000). The interview: From structured questions to negotiated text. In N. K. Denzin, & Y. S. Lincoln (Eds.), *Handbook of qualitative research* (2nd ed., pp. 645–672). Sage.

Fonteyn, M. E., Kuipers, B., & Grobe, S. J. (1993). A description of think aloud method and protocol analysis. *Qualitative Health Research*, 3(4): 430–441.

Fox, J. E. (2016). The science of usability testing. In *Proceedings of the 2015 Federal Committee on Statistical Methodology (FCSM) Research Conference*. Retrieved from https://nces.ed.gov/fcsm/pdf/C2_Fox_2015FCSM.pdf

Fox, S., & Fallows, D. (2003). Internet health resources: Health searches and email have become more commonplace, but there is room for improvement in searches and overall Internet access. *Pew Internet Research*. Retrieved from www.pewinternet.org/2003/07/16/internet-health-resources

Fox, S., & Rainie, L. (2000). The online health care revolution: How the web helps Americans take better care of themselves. In *Pew internet & American life: Online life report*. Institute for Health Care Research and Policy.

Freeman, K. S., & Spyridakis, J. H. (2004). An examination of factors that affect the credibility of online health information. *Technical Communication*, 51(2), 239–263.

Gale, N. K., Heath, G., Cameron, E., Rashid, S., & Redwood, S. (2013). Using the framework method for the analysis of qualitative data in multi-disciplinary health research. *BMC Medical Research Methodology*, 13(1), 117. https://doi.org/10.1186/1471-2288-13-117

Gangwar, H., Date, H., & Raoot, A. D. (2014). Review on IT adoption: Insights from recent technologies. *Journal of Enterprise Information Management*, 27(4), 488–502. https://doi.org/10.1108/JEIM-08-2012-0047

Gans, H. J. (1999). Participant observation in the era of "ethnography." *Journal of Contemporary Ethnography*, 28, 540–548.

gazepoint. (n.d.). gazepoint website. Retrieved from www.gazept.com

Georgsson, M., & Staggers, N. (2016). Quantifying usability: An evaluation of a diabetes mHealth system on effectiveness, efficiency, and satisfaction metrics with associated user characteristics. *Journal of the American Medical Informatics Association*, 23(1), 5–11. https://doi.org/10.1093/jamia/ocv099

Gerhardt-Powals, J. (1996). Cognitive engineering principles for enhancing human–computer performance. *International Journal of Human–Computer Interaction*, 8(2), 189–211. https://doi.org/10.1080/10447319609526147

Gibbons, M. C., Lowry, S. Z., & Patterson, E. S. (2014). Applying human factors principles to mitigate usability issues related to embedded assumptions in health information technology design. *JMIR Human Factors*, 1(1), e3. https://doi.org/10.2196/humanfactors.3524

Gigerenzer, G., & Goldstein, D. G. (1996). Reasoning the fast and frugal way: Models of bounded rationality. *Psychological Review*, 103(4), 650–669.

Golafshani, N. (2003). Understanding reliability and validity in qualitative research. *The Qualitative Report*, 8(4), 597–607. https://doi.org/10.46743/2160-3715/2003.1870

Goldberg, J. H. (2000). Eye movement-based interface evaluation: What can and cannot be assessed? *Proceedings of the Human Factors and Ergonomics Society Annual Meeting*, 44(37), 625–628. https://doi.org/10.1177/154193120004403721

Goldberg, L., Lide, B., Lowry, S., Massett, H. A., O'Connell, T., Preece, J., Quesenbery, W., & Shneiderman, B. (2011). Usability and accessibility in consumer health informatics. *American Journal of Preventive Medicine*, 40(5), S187–S197. https://doi.org/10.1016/j.amepre.2011.01.009

Goldeberg, J. H., & Wichansky, A. M. (2003). Eye tracking in usability evaluation: A practitioner's guide. In J. Hyönä, R. Radach, & H. Deubel (Eds.), *The Mind's Eyes: Cognitive and Applied Aspects of Eye Movements* (pp. 493–516). Elsevier.

González, M., Masip, L., Granollers, A., & Oliva, M. (2009). Quantitative analysis in a heuristic evaluation experiment. *Advances in Engineering Software*, 40(12), 1271–1278. https://doi.org/10.1016/j.advengsoft.2009.01.027

Google Forms. Available from https://docs.google.com/forms

Gould, J. D., & Lewis, C. (1985). Designing for usability: Key principles and what designers think. *Communications of the ACM*, 28(3), 300–311. https://doi.org/10.1145/3166.3170

Granollers, T. (2022, March 19). Beyond Nielsen's list (combining Nielsen's and Tog's). *UX Heuristics*. Retrieved from https://uxheuristics.net/heuristics/beyond-nielsen-s-list-combining-nielsens-and-togs

Gray, N. J., Klein, J. D., Noyce, P. R., Sesselberg, T. S., & Cantrill, J. A. (2005). The Internet: A window on adolescent health literacy. *The Journal of Adolescent Health*, 37(3), 243. https://doi.org/10.1016/j.jadohealth.2004.08.023

Gray, W.D., & Salzman, M. C. (1998). Damaged merchandise? A review of experiments that compare usability evaluation methods. *Human–Computer Interaction*, 13, 203–262.

Greenhalgh, T., Procter, R., Wherton, J., & Sugarhood, P. (2012). The organising vision for telehealth and telecare: discourse analysis. *BMJ Open*, 2(4), e001574. https://doi.org/10.1136/bmjopen-2012-001574

Grudin, J. (1992). Utility and usability: Research issues and development contexts. *Interacting with Computers*, 4(2), 209–217. https://doi.org/10.1016/0953-5438(92)90005-Z

Guba, E. G., & Lincoln, Y. S. (1996). Competing paradigms in qualitative research. In N.K. Denzin & Y.S. Lincoln (Eds.), *The Sage Handbook of Qualitative Research* (pp. 105–117). Sage.

Hajesmaeel-Gohari, S., & Bahaadinbeigy, K. (2021). The most used questionnaires for evaluating telemedicine services. *BMC Medical Informatics and Decision Making*, 21(1), 36. https://doi.org/10.1186/s12911-021-01407-y

Hamad, E. O., Savundranayagam, M. Y., Holmes, J. D., Kinsella, E. A., & Johnson, A. M. (2016). Toward a mixed-methods research approach to content analysis in the digital age: The combined content-analysis model and its applications to health care Twitter feeds. *Journal of Medical Internet Research*, 18(3), e5391. https://doi.org/10.2196/jmir.5391

Hammond, K. R. (1998). Judgment and decision making in dynamic tasks. *Information Decision Technologies*, 14, 3–14.

Harte, R., Glynn, L., Rodríguez-Molinero, A., Baker, P. M., Scharf, T., Quinlan, L. R., & ÓLaighin, G. (2017). A human-centered design methodology to enhance the usability, human factors, and user experience of connected health systems: A three-phase methodology. *JMIR Human Factors*, 4(1), e8. https://doi.org/10.2196/humanfactors.5443

Hassenzahl, M., Burmester, M., & Koller, F. (2003). AttrakDiff: Ein Fragebogen zur Messung wahrgenommener hedonischer und pragmatischer Qualität. B.G. Teubner. Retrieved from http://dl.gi.de/handle/20.500.12116/7308

Health Information Technology for Economic and Clinical Health (HITECH) Act, Vol. 74, No. 209 (October 30, 2009).

Hendriks, Y., Peek, S., Kaptein, M., & Bongers, I. (2022). Process and information needs when searching for and selecting apps for smoking cessation: Qualitative study using contextual inquiry. *JMIR Human Factors*, 9(2), e32628. https://doi.org/10.2196/32628

Henneman, P. L., Fisher, D. L., Henneman, E. A., Pham, T. A., Mei, Y. Y., Talati, R., Nathanson, B. H., & Roche, J. (2008). Providers do not verify patient identity during computer order entry. *Academic Emergency Medicine*, 15(7), 641–648. https://doi.org/10.1111/j.1553-2712.2008.00148.x

Hesse, B. W., Nelson, D. E., Kreps, G. L., Croyle, R. T., Arora, N. K., Rimer, B. K., … Viswanath, K. (2005). Trust and sources of health information: The impact of the internet and its implications for health care providers: Findings from the first Health Information National Trends Survey. *Archives of Internal Medicine*, 165, 2618–2624.

Hibbard, J. H., & Peters, E. (2003). Supporting informed consumer health care decisions: Data presentation approaches that facilitate the use of information in choice. *Annual Review of Public Health*, 24(1), 413–433.

Hibbard, J. H., Slovic, P., & Jewett, J. J. (1997). Informing consumer decisions in health care: implications from decision making research. *Milbank Quarterly*, 75, 395–414.

Hirani, S. P., Rixon, L., Beynon, M., Cartwright, M., Cleanthous, S., Selva, A., Sanders, C., & Newman, S. P. (2017). Quantifying beliefs regarding telehealth: Development of the Whole Systems Demonstrator Service User Technology Acceptability Questionnaire. *Journal of Telemedicine and Telecare*, 23(4), 460–469. https://doi.org/10.1177/1357633X1 6649531

Holsti, O. R. (1969). *Content analysis for the social sciences and humanities*. Addison-Wesley.

Hornbæk, K. (2006). Current practice in measuring usability: Challenges to usability studies and research. *International Journal of Human–Computer Studies*, 64(2), 79–102. https://doi. org/10.1016/j.ijhcs.2005.06.002

Horsky, J., & Ramelson, H. Z. (2016). Development of a cognitive framework of patient record summary review in the formative phase of user-centered design. *Journal of Biomedical Information*, 64, 147–157.

Høstgaard, A. M., Bertelsen, P., & Nøhr, C. (2011). Methods to identify, study and understand end-user participation in HIT development. *BMC Medical Informatics and Decision Making*, 11(1), 57. https://doi.org/10.1186/1472-6947-11-57

Howell, K. E. (2013). *An introduction to the philosophy of methodology*. Sage.

Hsieh, H.-F., & Shannon, S. E. (2005). Three approaches to qualitative content analysis. *Qualitative Health Research*, 15(9), 1277–1288. https://doi.org/10.1177/104973230 5276687

Hsiu-Fang, H., & Shannon, S. E. (2005). Three approaches to qualitative content analysis. *Qualitative Health Research*, 15(9), 1277–1288. https://doi.org/10.1177/104973230 5276687

Hsu, W., Chiang, C., & Yang, S. (2014). The effect of individual factors on health behaviors among college students: The mediating effects of eHealth literacy. *Journal of Medical Internet Research*, 16(12), e287. https://doi.org/10.2196/jmir.3542

Hughes, M. (1999). Rigor in usability testing. *Technical Communication: Journal of the Society for Technical Communication*, 46(4), 488–494.

Hung, M., Conrad, J., Hon, S. D., Cheng, C., Franklin, J. D., & Tang, P. (2013). Uncovering patterns of technology use in consumer health informatics. *Computational Statistics*, 5(6), 432–447. https://doi.org/10.1002/wics.1276

Impicciatore, P., Pandolfini, C., Casella, N., & Bonati, M. (1997). Reliability of health information for the public on the World Wide Web: Systematic survey of advice on managing fever in children at home. *BMJ Clinical Research*, 314(7098), 1875–1879. https://doi.org/ 10.1136/bmj.314.7098.1875

Indria, D., Alajlani, M., & Fraser, H. (2020). Clinicians' perceptions of a telemedicine system: A mixed method study of Makassar City, Indonesia. *BMC Medical Informatics and Decision Making*, 20, 233. https://doi.org/10.1186/s12911-020-01234-7

International Organization for Standardization (ISO). (1991). 9126:1991—*Software engineering: Product quality*. Geneva: ISO/IEC.

International Organization for Standardization (ISO). (2001). 9126-1:2001—*Software engineering: Product quality*. Geneva: ISO/IEC.

International Organization for Standardization (ISO) (2017). 25010:2011—*Systems and software engineering: Systems and software quality requirements and evaluation (SQuaRE) system and software quality models*. Geneva: ISO/IEC.

International Organization for Standardization (ISO). (2018). 9241-11:2018(en)—*Ergonomics of human–system interaction, Part 11—Usability: Definitions and concepts.* Geneva: ISO/IEC.

International Organization for Standardization (ISO) (2019). 9241-210:2019—*Ergonomics of human–system interaction, Part 210: Human-centred design for interactive systems.* Geneva: ISO/IEC.

Islam, M. N., Karim, M. M., Inan, T. T., & Islam, A. K. M. N. (2020). Investigating usability of mobile health applications in Bangladesh. *BMC Medical Informatics and Decision Making*, 20(1), 19. https://doi.org/10.1186/s12911-020-1033-3

J. Sauro & J. R. Lewis, personal communication, January 27, 2023.

Jacob, R. J. K., & Karn, K. S. (2003). Eye tracking in human–computer interaction and usability research: Ready to deliver the promises. In J. Hyön, R. Radach, & H. Deubel (Eds.), *The mind's eye: Cognitive and applied aspects of eye movement research* (pp. 573–605). North-Holland.

Jalil, S., Myers, T., Atkinson, I., & Soden, M. (2019). Complementing a clinical trial with human–computer interaction: Patients' user experience with telehealth. *JMIR Human Factors*, 6(2), e9481. https://doi.org/10.2196/humanfactors.9481

Jarrahi, M. H., Goray, C., Zirker, S., & Zhang, Y. (2021). Digital diaries as a research method for capturing practices in situ. In M. H. Jarrahi, C. Goray, S. Zirker, & Y. Zhang (Eds.), *Research methods for digital work and organization* (pp. 107–129). Oxford University Press. https://doi.org/10.1093/oso/9780198860679.003.0006

Jaspers, M., Steen, T., Bos, C., & Geenen, M. (2004). The think aloud method: A guide to user interface design. *International Journal of Medical Informatics*, 73(11–12), 781–795. https://doi.org/10.1016/j.ijmedinf.2004.08.003

Jeffries, R. (1994). Usability problem reports: Helping evaluators communicate effectively with developers. In J. Nielsen, & R. L. Mack (Eds.), *Usability inspection methods* (pp. 274–291). John Wiley & Sons.

Jeffries, R., Miller, J. R., Wharton, C., & Uyeda, K. (1991). User interface evaluation in the real world: A comparison of four techniques. In *Proceedings of the SIGCHI Conference on Human Factors in Computing Systems Reaching through Technology—CHI '91*, 119–124. https://doi.org/10.1145/108844.108862

Jetha, A., Faulkner, G., Gorczynski, P., Arbour-Nicitopoulos, K., & Ginis, K. A. M. (2011). Physical activity and individuals with spinal cord injury: Accuracy and quality of information on the internet. *Disability and Health Journal*, 4(2), 112–120.

Johnson, C. M., Johnson, T. R., & Zhang, J. (2005). A user-centered framework for redesigning health care interfaces. *Journal of Biomedical Informatics*, 38(1), 75–87.

Johnson, J. L., Adkins, D., & Chauvin, S. (2020). A review of the quality indicators of rigor in qualitative research. *American Journal of Pharmaceutical Education*, 84(1), 7120. https://doi.org/10.5688/ajpe7120

Johnson, R. B., Onwuegbuzie, A. J., & Turner, L. A. (2007). Toward a definition of mixed methods research. *Journal of Mixed Methods Research*, 1(2), 112–133. https://doi.org/10.1177/1558689806298224

Jokela, T., Koivumaa, J., Pirkola, J., Salminen, P., & Kantola, N. (2006). Methods for quantitative usability requirements: A case study on the development of the user interface of a mobile phone. *Personal and Ubiquitous Computing*, 10(6), 345–355. https://doi.org/10.1007/s00779-005-0050-7

Jones, J. A. (1989). The verbal protocol: A research technique for nursing. *Journal of Advanced Nursing*, 14, 1062–1070.

Kaipio, J., Lääveri, T., Hyppönen, H., Vainiomäki, S., Reponen, J., Kushniruk, A., Borycki, E., & Vänskä, J. (2017). Usability problems do not heal by themselves: National survey on physicians' experiences with EHRs in Finland. *International Journal of Medical Informatics*, 97, 266–281. https://doi.org/10.1016/j.ijmedinf.2016.10.010

Katusiime, B., Corlett, S., Reeve, J., & Krska, J. (2016). Measuring medicine-related experiences from the patient perspective: A systematic review. *Patient Related Outcome Measures*, 7, 157–171. https://doi.org/10.2147/PROM.S102198

Kayyali, R., Hesso, I., Ejiko, E., & Nabhani Gebara, S. (2017). A qualitative study of telehealth patient information leaflets (TILs): Are we giving patients enough information? *BMC Health Services Research*, 17(1), 362. https://doi.org/10.1186/s12913-017-2257-5

Kellermann, A. L., & Jones, S. S. (2013). What it will take to achieve the as-yet-unfulfilled promises of health Information Technology. *Health Affairs*, 32(1), 63–68. https://doi.org/10.1377/hlthaff.2012.0693

Khairat, S., Coleman, C., Newlin, T., Rand, V., Ottmar, P., Bice, T., & Carson, S. S. (2019). A mixed-methods evaluation framework for electronic health records usability studies. *Journal of Biomedical Informatics*, 94, 103175. https://doi.org/10.1016/j.jbi.2019.103175

Khairat, S., Coleman, C., Ottmar, P., Jayachander, D. I., Bice, T., & Carson, S. S. (2020). Association of electronic health record use with physician fatigue and efficiency. *JAMA Network Open*, 3(6), e207385. https://doi.org/10.1001/jamanetworkopen.2020.7385

Khairat, S., Zalla, L., Gartland, A., & Seashore, C. (2021). Association between proficiency and efficiency in electronic health records among pediatricians at a major academic health system. *Frontiers in Digital Health*, 3, 689646. https://doi.org/10.3389/fdgth.2021.689646

Khajouei, R., de Jongh, D., & Jaspers, M. W. M. (2009). Usability evaluation of a computerized physician order Entry for Medication Ordering. *Studies in Health Technology Information*, 150, 532–536.

Khajouei, R., & Jaspers, M. W. M. (2008). CPOE system design aspects and their qualitative effect on usability. *Studies in Health Technology Information*, 136, 309–314.

Khajouei, R., Zahiri Esfahani, M., & Jahani, Y. (2017). Comparison of heuristic and cognitive walkthrough usability evaluation methods for evaluating health information systems. *Journal of the American Medical Informatics Association*, 24(e1), e55–e60. https://doi.org/10.1093/jamia/ocw100

Khaled, R., Biddle, R., Noble, J., Barr, P., & Fischer, R. (2006). Persuasive interaction for collectivist cultures. In *Proceedings of the 7th Australasian User Interface Conference*. 50, 73–80.

Khowaja, K., & Al-Thani, D. (2020). New checklist for the heuristic evaluation of mHealth apps (HE4EH): Development and usability study. *JMIR MHealth and UHealth*, 8(10), e20353. https://doi.org/10.2196/20353

Kieras, D. (2004). GOMS models and task analysis. In D. Diaper & N. A. Stanton (Eds.), *The handbook of task analysis for human-computer interaction* (pp. 83–116). Lawrence Erlbaum.

Kinzie, M. B., Cohn, W. F., Julian, M. F., & Knaus, W. A. (2002). A user-centered model for web site design: Needs assessment, user interface design, and rapid prototyping. *Journal of the American Medical Informatics Association*, 9(4), 320–330. https://doi.org/10.1197/jamia.m0822

Krawiec, Ł., & Dudycz, H. (2020). A comparison of heuristics applied for studying the usability of websites. *Procedia Computer Science*, 176, 3571–3580. https://doi.org/10.1016/j.procs.2020.09.029

Krefting, L. (1991). Rigor in qualitative research: The assessment of trustworthiness. *The American Journal of Occupational Therapy*, 45(3), 214–222.

Krieger, N., & Bassett, M. (1986). The health of black folk: Disease, class, and ideology in science. *Monthly Review*, 38, 74–85.

Krippendorff, K. (1980). *Content analysis: An introduction to its methodology*. Sage.

Krippendorff, K. (2004). *Content analysis: An introduction to its methodology* (2nd ed.). Sage.

Krippendorff, K. (2011). Computing Krippendorff's alpha-reliability. University of Pennsylvania. Retrieved from https://repository.upenn.edu/asc_papers/43

Krueger, R. A. (1998). *Developing questions for focus groups.* Sage.

Krueger, R. A., & Casey, M. A. (2009). *Focus groups: A practical guide for applied research* (4th ed). Sage.

Kuhn, T. S. (1962). *The structure of scientific revolutions* (3rd ed). University of Chicago Press.

Kushniruk, A. W. (2001). Analysis of complex decision-making processes in health care: Cognitive approaches to health informatics. *Journal of Biomedical Informatics*, 34(5), 365–376.

Kushniruk, A. W. (2002). Evaluation in the design of health information systems: Application of approaches emerging from usability engineering. *Computers in Biology and Medicine*, 32, 141–149.

Kushniruk, A., Beuscart-Zéphir, M.-C., Grzes, A., Borycki, E., & Kannry, L. W. (2010). Increasing the safety of healthcare information systems through improved procurement: Toward a framework for selection of safe healthcare systems. *Healthcare Quarterly*, 13. Retrieved from www.longwoods.com/content/21967/healthcare-quarterly/increasing-the-safety-of-healthcare-information-systems-through-improved-procurement-toward-a-frame

Kushniruk, A. W., & Borycki, E. M. (2015). Development of a video coding scheme for analyzing the usability and usefulness of health information systems. In E.M. Borycki, A.W. Kushnirui, C.E. Kuziemsky, & C. Nohr (Eds.), *Context sensitive health informatics: Many places, many users, many contexts, many uses* (pp. 68–73). IOS Press. https://doi.org/10.3233/978-1-61499-574-6-68

Kushniruk, A., Borycki, E., Kitson, N., & Kannry, J. (2019a). Development of a video coding scheme focused on socio-technical aspects of human–computer interaction in healthcare. *Studies in Health Technology and Informatics*, 257, 236–243.

Kushniruk, A. W., Borycki, E. M., Kuwata, S., & Ho, F. (2008). Emerging approaches to evaluating the usability of health information systems. In A. W. Kushniruk, & E. M. Borycki (Eds.), *Human, social, and organizational aspects of health information systems* (pp. 1–22). IGI Global.

Kushniruk, A. W., Kan, M.-Y., McKeown, K., Klavans, J., Jordan, D., LaFlamme, M., & Patel, V. L. (2002). Usability evaluation of an experimental text summarization system and three search engines: Implications for the reengineering of health care interfaces. In *Proceedings of the AMIA Symposium*, 420–424.

Kushniruk, A. W., Kaufman, D. R., Patel, V. L., Lévesque, Y., & Lottin, P. (1996). Assessment of a computerized patient record system: A cognitive approach to evaluating medical technology. *M.D. Computing: Computers in Medical Practice*, 13(5), 406–415.

Kushniruk, A. W., Monkman, H., Kitson, N., & Borycki, E. M. (2019b). Development of a video coding scheme for understanding human–computer interaction and clinical decision making. *Studies in Health Technology and Informatics*, 265, 80–85. https://doi.org/10.3233/SHTI190142

Kushniruk, A., & Nøhr, C. (2016). Participatory design, user involvement and health IT evaluation. *Studies in Health Technology and Informatics*, 222, 139–151. Retrieved from https://pubmed.ncbi.nlm.nih.gov/27198099

Kushniruk, A., Nohr, C., Jensen, S., & Borycki, E. M. (2013). From usability testing to clinical simulations: Bringing context into the design and evaluation of usable and safe health information technologies: Contribution of the IMIA Human Factors Engineering for Healthcare Informatics Working Group. *Yearbook of Medical Informatics*, 22(1), 78–85. https://doi.org/10.1055/s-0038-1638836

Kushniruk, A. W., & Patel, V. L. (2004). Cognitive and usability engineering methods for the evaluation of clinical information systems. *Journal of Biomedical Informatics*, 37(1), 56–76. https://doi.org/10.1016/j.jbi.2004.01.003

Kushniruk, A. W., & Patel, V. L. (2005). Cognitive approaches to the evaluation of healthcare information systems. In J. G. Anderson, & C. E. Aydin (Eds.), *Health Informatics* (pp. 144–173). Springer.

Kushniruk, A. W., Patel, C., Patel, V. L., & Cimino, J. J. (2001). "Televaluation" of clinical information systems: An integrative approach to assessing web-based systems. *International Journal of Medical Informatics*, 61, 45–70.

Kushniruk, A. W., Patel, V. L., & Cimino, J. J. (1997). Usability testing in medical informatics: Cognitive approaches to evaluation of information systems and user interfaces. In *Proceedings of Conference of the American Medical Informatics Association: AMIA Fall Symposium*, 218–222. Retrieved from www.ncbi.nlm.nih.gov/pmc/articles/PMC2233486

Kutner, M., Greenberg, E., Jin Y, Paulsen, C., & American Institutes for Research. (2006). *The Health Literacy of America's Adults Results From the 2003 National Assessment of Adult Literacy* (NCES 2006–483). National Center for Education. Retrieved from http://files.eric.ed.gov/fulltext/ED493284.pdf

Langbecker, D., Caffery, L. J., Gillespie, N., & Smith, A. C. (2017). Using survey methods in telehealth research: A practical guide. *Journal of Telemedicine and Telecare*, 23(9), 770–779. https://doi.org/10.1177/1357633X17721814

Lee, K., Hoti, K., Hughes, J. D., & Emmerton, L. (2014). Dr Google and the consumer: A qualitative study exploring the navigational needs and online health information-seeking behaviors of consumers with chronic health conditions. *Journal of Medical Internet Research*, 16(12), e262. https://doi.org/10.2196/jmir.3706

Lee, K., Hoti, K., Hughes, J. D., & Emmerton, L. M. (2015). Consumer use of "Dr Google": A survey on health information-seeking behaviors and navigational needs. *Journal of Medical Internet Research*, 17(12), e288. https://doi.org/10.2196/jmir.4345

Leprohon, J., & Patel, V. L. (1995). Decision strategies in emergency telephone triage. *Medical Decision Making*, 15(3), 240–253.

Leslie, M., Paradis, E., Gropper, M. A., Kitto, S., Reeves, S., & Pronovost, P. (2017). An ethnographic study of health information technology use in three intensive care units. *Health Services Research*, 52(4), 1330–1348. https://doi.org/10.1111/1475-6773.12466

Lewis, J. R. (1991). Psychometric evaluation of an after-scenario questionnaire for computer usability studies: The ASQ. *ACM SIGCHI Bulletin*, 23(1), 78–81. https://doi.org/10.1145/122672.122692

Lewis, J. R. (1992). Psychometric evaluation of the post-study system usability questionnaire: The PSSUQ. *Proceedings of the Human Factors and Ergonomics Society Annual Meeting*, 36(16), 1259–1260.

Lewis, J. R. (1995). IBM computer usability satisfaction questionnaires: Psychometric evaluation and instructions for use. *International Journal of Human–Computer Interaction*, 7(1), 57–78. https://doi.org/10.1080/10447319509526110

Lewis, J. R. (2002). Psychometric evaluation of the PSSUQ using data from five years of usability studies. *International Journal of Human–Computer Interaction*, 14(3–4), 463–488. https://doi.org/10.1080/10447318.2002.9669130

Lewis, J. R. (2006). Usability testing. In G. Salvendy (Ed.), *Handbook of human factors and ergonomics* (pp. 1275–1316). John Wiley & Sons.

Lewis, J. R., & Sauro, J. (2009). The factor structure of the System Usability Scale. In M. Kurosu (Ed.), *Human centered design* (Vol. 5619, pp. 94–103). Springer. https://doi.org/10.1007/978-3-642-02806-9_12

Lewis, J. R., & Sauro, J. (2018). Item benchmarks for the System Usability Scale. *Journal of Usability Studies*, 13(3), 158–167.

Li, A. C., Kannry, J. L., Kushniruk, A., Chrimes, D., McGinn, T. G., Edonyabo, D., & Mann, D. M. (2012). Integrating usability testing and think-aloud protocol analysis with "near-live" clinical simulations in evaluating clinical decision support. *International Journal of Medical Informatics*, 81(11), 761–772. https://doi.org/10.1016/j.ijmedinf.2012.02.009

Li, L. C., Adam, P. M., Townsend, A. F., Lacaille, D., Yousefi, C., Stacey, D., Gromala, D., Shaw, C. D., Tugwell, P., & Backman, C. L. (2013). Usability testing of ANSWER: A web-based methotrexate decision aid for patients with rheumatoid arthritis. *BMC Medical Informatics and Decision Making*, 13, 131. https://doi.org/10.1186/1472-6947-13-131

Lincoln, Y. S., & Guba, E. G. (1985). *Naturalistic inquiry*. Beverly Hills, CA: Sage.

Long, T., & Johnson, M. (2000). Rigour, reliability and validity in qualitative research. *Clinical Effectiveness in Nursing*, 4(1), 30–37.

Lowry, S., Quinn, M., Ramaiah, M., Schumacher, R., Patterson, E., & North, R. (2012). *Technical evaluation, testing and validation of the usability of electronic health records, NIST Interagency/Internal Report (NISTIR) (NISTIR 7804)*. National Institute of Standards and Technology. https://doi.org/10.6028/NIST.IR.7804

Lu, J., Yao, J., & Yu, C. (2005). Personal innovativeness, social influences and adoption of wireless internet services via mobile technology. *The Journal of Strategic Information Systems*, 14(3), 245–268.

Luger, T. M., Houston, T. K., & Suls, J. (2014). Older adult experience of online diagnosis: Results from a scenario-based think-aloud protocol. *Journal of Medical Internet Research*, 16(1), e16. https://doi.org/10.2196/jmir.2924

Lundgrén-Laine, H., & Salanterä, S. (2010). Think-aloud technique and protocol analysis in clinical decision-making research. *Qualitative Health Research*, 20(4), 565–575.

Lyles, C. R., Sarkar, U., & Osborn, C. Y. (2014). Getting a technology-based diabetes intervention ready for primetime: A review of usability testing studies. *Current Diabetes Reports*, 14(10), 534. https://doi.org/10.1007/s11892-014-0534-9

Macias, W., Lee, M., & Cunningham, N. (2018). Inside the mind of the online health information searcher using think-aloud protocol. *Health Communication*, 33(12), 1482–1493. https://doi.org/10.1080/10410236.2017.1372040

Maher, C., Hadfield, M., Hutchings, M., & de Eyto, A. (2018). Ensuring rigor in qualitative data analysis: A design research approach to coding combining NVivo with traditional material methods. *International Journal of Qualitative Methods*, 17(1), 1609406918786362. https://doi.org/10.1177/1609406918786362

Main, C., Moxham, T., Wyatt, J. C., Kay, J., Anderson, R., & Stein, K. (2010). Computerised decision support systems in order communication for diagnostic, screening or monitoring test ordering: Systematic reviews of the effects and cost-effectiveness of systems. *Health Technology Assessment*, 14(48), 1–227. https://doi.org/10.3310/hta14480

Mann, D. M., Chokshi, S. K., & Kushniruk, A. (2018). Bridging the gap between academic research and pragmatic needs in usability: A hybrid approach to usability evaluation of health care information systems. *JMIR Human Factors*, 5(4), e10721. https://doi.org/10.2196/10721

Maramba, I., Chatterjee, A., & Newman, C. (2019). Methods of usability testing in the development of eHealth applications: A scoping review. *International Journal of Medical Informatics*, 126, 95–104. https://doi.org/10.1016/j.ijmedinf.2019.03.018

Marco-Ruiz, L., Bønes, E., Asunción, E. d., Gabarron, E., Aviles-Solis, J. C., Lee, E., ... Bellika, J. G. (2017). Combining multivariate statistics and the think-aloud protocol to assess Human-Computer Interaction barriers in symptom checkers. *Journal of Biomedical Informatics*, 74, 104–122.

Marquart, F. (2017). Methodological rigor in quantitative research. In J. Matthes, C. S. Davis, & R. F. Potter (Eds.), *The International Encyclopedia of Communication Research Methods* (pp. 1–9). Wiley. https://doi.org/10.1002/9781118901731.iecrm0221

Martínez-Mesa, J., González-Chica, D. A., Bastos, J. L., Bonamigo, R. R., & Duquia, R. P. (2014). Sample size: how many participants do I need in my research? *Anais Brasileiros de Dermatologia*, 89(4), 609–615. https://doi.org/10.1590/abd1806-4841.20143705

Mason, M. (2010). Sample Size and Saturation in PhD Studies Using Qualitative Interviews. Methods for Qualitative Management Research in the Context of Social Systems, 11(3). https://doi.org/10.17169/FQS-11.3.1428

MAXQDA. (n.d.). All-in-one Qualitative Data Analysis Software. MAXQDA. Retrieved from www.maxqda.com/

Mayhew, D. J. (1999). *The usability engineering lifecycle: A practitioner's handbook for user interface design*. Morgan Kaufmann Publishers.

Mays, N., & Pope, C. (1995). Rigour and qualitative research. *BMJ: The British Medical Journal*, 311, 109–112.

McCambridge, J., Witton, J., & Elbourne, D. R. (2014). Systematic review of the Hawthorne effect: new concepts are needed to study research participation effects. *Journal of Clinical Epidemiology*, 67(3), 267–277.

McHugh M. L. (2012). Interrater reliability: the kappa statistic. *Biochemia medica*, 22(3), 276–282.

McKnight, H., Choudhury, V., & Kacmarc, C. (2002). The impact of initial consumer trust on intentions to transact with a web site: a trust building model. *Journal of Strategic Information Systems*, 11(3-4), 297–323.

Meloncon, L. (2016). Patient Experience Design: Technical Communication's Role in Patient Health Information and Education. *Intercom*. January. Retrieved from www.stc.org/inter com/2016/02/patient-experience-design-technical-communications-role-in-patient-hea lth-information-and-education/

Meloncon, L. (2017). Patient Experience Design: Expanding Usability Methodologies for Healthcare. *Communication Design Quarterly*. 5(2), 19–28.

Meyrick, J. (2006). What is Good Qualitative Research?: A First Step towards a Comprehensive Approach to Judging Rigour/Quality. *Journal of Health Psychology*, 11(5), 799–808. https://doi.org/10.1177/1359105306066643

Milward, J., Deluca, P., Drummond, C., Watson, R., Dunne, J., & Kimergård, A. (2017). Usability Testing of the BRANCH Smartphone App Designed to Reduce Harmful Drinking in Young Adults. *JMIR mHealth and uHealth*, 5(8), e109. doi:10.2196/mhealth.7836

Mirel, B. (2004). *Interaction design for complex problem solving: Developing useful and usable software*. Elsevier.

Mishra, S. B., & Alok, S. (2017). *Handbook of Research Methodology: A Compendium for Scholars & Researchers*. Educreation Publishing.

Monkman, H., & Kushniruk, A. (2013a). A health literacy and usability heuristic evaluation of a mobile consumer health application. *Studies in Health Technology and Informatics*, 192, 724–728.

Monkman, H., & Kushniruk, A. (2013b). Applying usability methods to identify health literacy issues: an example using a Personal Health Record. *Studies in health technology and informatics*, 183, 179–185. doi:10.3233/978-1-61499-203-5-179

Monkman, H., & Kushniruk, A. (2015). eHealth literacy issues, constructs, models, and methods for health information technology design and evaluation. *Knowledge Management & E-Learning: An International Journal*, 7(4), Article 4.

Moran, K. (2016, December 11). Reading Content on Mobile Devices. *Nielsen Norman Group*. Retrieved from www.nngroup.com/articles/mobile-content/

Morgan, D. L. (1998). Practical Strategies for Combining Qualitative and Quantitative Methods: Applications to Health Research. *Qualitative Health Research*, 8(3), 362–376. https://doi.org/10.1177/104973239800800307

Morgan-Trimmer, S., & Wood, F. (2016). Ethnographic methods for process evaluations of complex health behaviour interventions. *Trials*, 17(1), 232. https://doi.org/10.1186/s13063-016-1340-2

Morony, S., McCaffery, K. J., Kirkendall, S., Jansen, J., & Webster, A. C. (2017). Health Literacy Demand of Printed Lifestyle Patient Information Materials Aimed at People With Chronic Kidney Disease: Are Materials Easy to Understand and Act On and Do They Use Meaningful Visual Aids?. *Journal of Health Communication*, 22(2), 163–170. https://doi.org/10.1080/10810730.2016.1258744

Morse, J. M. (1994). Designing qualitative research. In N. K. Denzin & Y. S. Lincoln (Eds.), *Handbook of qualitative inquiry* (pp. 220–235). Sage.

Morse, J. M. (2000). Determining Sample Size. *Qualitative Health Research*, 10(1), 3–5. https://doi.org/10.1177/104973200129118183\

Mortari, L. (2015). Reflectivity in Research Practice: An Overview of Different Perspectives. *International Journal of Qualitative Methods*, 14(5), 1609406915618045. https://doi.org/10.1177/1609406915618045

Murray-Torres, T., Casarella, A., Bollini, M., Wallace, F., Avidan, M. S., & Politi, M. C. (2019). Anesthesiology Control Tower—Feasibility Assessment to Support Translation (ACTFAST): Mixed-Methods Study of a Novel Telemedicine-Based Support System for the Operating Room. *JMIR Human Factors*, 6(2), e12155. https://doi.org/10.2196/12155

N. K. Gale, personal communication, August 16, 2021.

Nassar, V. (2012). Common criteria for usability review. *Work*, 41, 1053–1057. https://doi.org/10.3233/WOR-2012-0282-1053

Nelson, S. D., LaFleur, J., Del Fiol, G., Evans, R. S., & Weir C. R. (2015). Reading and Writing: Qualitative Analysis of Pharmacists' Use of the EHR when Preparing for Team Rounds. *AMIA Annual Symposium Proceedings*, 943–952. Retrieved from https://europepmc.org/article/pmc/pmc4765606#b34-2246265

Nielsen J. (2000, March 19). Why You Only Need to Test with 5 Users. *Nielsen Norman Group*. Retrieved from www.nngroup.com/articles/why-you-only-need-to-test-with-5-users

Nielsen, J. (1989). Usability engineering at a discount. *Proceedings of the Third International Conference on Human-Computer Interaction on Designing and Using Human-Computer Interfaces and Knowledge Based Systems* (2nd ed.), 394–401.

Nielsen, J. (1992). Finding usability problems through heuristic evaluation. *Proceedings of the SIGCHI Conference on Human Factors in Computing Systems – CHI '92*, 373–380. https://doi.org/10.1145/142750.142834

Nielsen, J. (1993a). *Usability engineering*. Academic Press.

Nielsen, J. (1993b). Iterative user-interface design. *Computer*, 26(11), 32–41. https://doi.org/10.1109/2.241424

Nielsen, J. (1994a). Estimating the number of subjects needed for a thinking aloud test. International Journal of Human-Computer Studies, 41(3), 385–397. https://doi.org/10.1006/ijhc.1994.1065

Nielsen, J. (1994b). Heuristic evaluation. In Nielsen, J., and Mack, R.L. (Eds.), *Usability Inspection Methods* (pp. 25–62). John Wiley & Son.

Nielsen, J. (1995). Applying discount usability engineering. *IEEE Software*, 12(1), 98–100. https://doi.org/10.1109/52.363161

Nielsen, J. (2015, November 15). Legibility, Readability, and Comprehension: Making Users Read Your Words. Nielsen Norman Group. Retrieved from www.nngroup.com/articles/legibility-readability-comprehension

Nielsen, J. (2012). Usability 101: Introduction to Usability. Nielsen Norman Group. Retrieved from www.nngroup.com/articles/usability-101-introduction-to-usability

Nielsen, J., & Budiu, R. (2013). *Mobile usability*. New Riders.

Nielsen, J., & Landauer, T. K. (1993). A mathematical model of the finding of usability problems. In *Proceedings of the INTERACT '93 and CHI '93 Conference on Human Factors in Computing Systems (CHI '93)*. ACM, New York, NY, USA, 206–213.

Nielsen, J., & Mack, R. L. (Eds.). (1994). *Usability inspection methods*. Wiley.

Nielsen, J., & Molich, R. (1990). Heuristic evaluation of user interfaces. *Proceedings of the SIGCHI Conference on Human Factors in Computing Systems Empowering People – CHI '90*, 249–256. https://doi.org/10.1145/97243.97281

Noble, H., & Smith, J. (2015). Issues of validity and reliability in qualitative research. *Evidence Based Nursing*, 18(2), 34–35.

Norman, C. D., & Skinner, H. A. (2006). eHealth Literacy: Essential Skills for Consumer Health in a Networked World. *Journal of Medical Internet Research*, 8(2), e9. https://doi.org/10.2196/jmir.8.2.e9

Norman, D. (1988). *The Psychology of Everyday Things*. New York, NY: Basic Books.

Norman, D. A. (2013). The design of everyday things (Revised and expanded edition). Basic Books.

Norman, D. A., & Draper, S. W. (Eds.). (1986). *User centered system design: New perspectives on human-computer interaction*. Erlbaum.

Norman, D., & Nielsen, J. (n.d.). The Definition of User Experience (UX). Nielsen Norman Group. Retrieved from www.nngroup.com/articles/definition-user-experience/

O'Brien, H. L., & Toms, E. G. (2008). What is user engagement? A conceptual framework for defining user engagement with technology. *Journal of the American Society for Information Science and Technology*, 59(6), 938–955.

Office of the National Coordinator for Health Information Technology (ONC). (13, January 2010). *45 CFR Part 170—Health Information Technology Standards, Implementation Specifications, and Certification Criteria and Certification Programs for Health Information Technology*. (January, 13, 2010). Retrieved from www.ecfr.gov/current/title-45/subtitle-A/subchapter-D/part-170

Office of the National Coordinator for Health Information Technology (ONC). (2012). *Health Information Technology: Standards, Implementation Specifications, and Certification Criteria for Electronic Health Record Technology, 2014 edition*; Revisions to the Permanent Certification Program for Health Information Technology, Final Rule. 77 Fed. Reg. 171 (September 4, 2012). (to be codified at 45 C. F. R pts. 170). 54163–54292.

Oleinik, A., Popova, I., Kirdina, S., & Shatalova, T. (2014). On the choice of measures of reliability and validity in the content-analysis of texts. *Quality & Quantity*, 48(5), 2703–2718. https://doi.org/10.1007/s11135-013-9919-0

Olmsted-Hawala, E.L., Murphy, E.D., Hawala, S., & Ashenfelter, K.T. (2010). Think-aloud protocols: Analyzing three different think-aloud protocols with counts of verbalized frustrations in a usability study of an information-rich Web site. *2010 IEEE International Professional Communication Conference*, 60–66. https://ieeexplore.ieee.org/document/5529815/

Ooms, K., Coltekin, A., De Maeyer, P., Dupont, L., Fabrikant, S., Incoul, A., Kuhn, M., Slabbinck, H., Vansteenkiste, P., & Van der Haegen, L. (2015). Combining user logging with eye tracking for interactive and dynamic applications. *Behavior Research Methods*, 47(4), 977–993. https://doi.org/10.3758/s13428-014-0542-3

Or, C., & Tao, D. (2012). Usability Study of a Computer-Based Self-Management System for Older Adults with Chronic Diseases. *Journal of Medical Internet Research (JMIR) Research Protocols*, 1(2):e13. doi:10.2196/resprot.2184

Orji, R., & Mandryk, R. L. (2014). Developing culturally relevant design guidelines for encouraging healthy eating behavior. *International Journal of Human-Computer Studies*, 72, 207–223. https://doi.org/10.1016/j.ijhcs.2013.08.012

Pang, P. C.-I., Chang, S., Verspoor, K., & Pearce, J. (2016). Designing Health Websites Based on Users' Web-Based Information-Seeking Behaviors: A Mixed-Method Observational Study. *Journal of Medical Internet Research*, 18(6), e145. https://doi.org/10.2196/jmir.5661

Parmanto, B., Lewis, A. N., Jr, Graham, K. M., & Bertolet, M. H. (2016). Development of the Telehealth Usability Questionnaire (TUQ). *International Journal of Relerehabilitation*, 8(1), 3–10. https://doi.org/10.5195/ijt.2016.6196

Parmar, V. (2010). Disseminating maternal health information to rural women: A user centered design framework. *AMIA Annual Symposium Proceedings*, 592–596.

Patel, V. L, & Groen, G. J. (1986). Knowledge-based solution strategies in medical reasoning. *Cognitive Science*, 10(1), 91–116.

Patel, V. L., & Kushniruk, A. W. (1998). Interface design for health care environments: The role of cognitive science. *Proceedings of the AMIA Symposium*, 29–37. Retrieved from www.ncbi.nlm.nih.gov/pmc/articles/PMC2232103/

Petch, T. (2004). Content analysis of selected health information websites. *Action for Health*. http://summit.sfu.ca/item/335

Peters, K., & Halcomb, E. (2015). Interviews in qualitative research: A consideration of two very different issues in the use of interviews to collect research data. *Nurse Researcher*, 22(4), 6–7. https://doi.org/10.7748/nr.22.4.6.s2

Peute, L. W, Knijnenburg, S. L., Kremer, L. C., & Jaspers, M. W. M. (2015b). A concise and practical framework for the development and usability evaluation of patient information websites. *Applied Clinical Informatics*, 6, 383–399.

Peute, L. W. P., & Jaspers, M. W. M. (2007). The significance of a usability evaluation of an emerging laboratory order entry system. *International Journal of Medical Informatics*, 76(2–3), 157–168. https://doi.org/10.1016/j.ijmedinf.2006.06.003

Peute, L. W., de Keizer, N. F., & Jaspers, M. W. (2015a). The value of retrospective and concurrent think aloud in formative usability testing of a physician data query tool. *Journal of Biomedical Informatics*, 55, 1–10.

Polit, D. F., & Beck, C. T. (2010). Generalization in quantitative and qualitative research: Myths and strategies. *International Journal of Nursing Studies*, 47(11), 1451–1458. https://doi.org/10.1016/j.ijnurstu.2010.06.004

Polson, P. G. & Lewis, C. H. (1990). Theory-based design for easily learned interfaces. *Human–Computer Interaction*, 5(2–3), 191–220. https://doi.org/10.1080/07370024.1990.9667154

Polson, P. G., Lewis, C., Rieman, J., & Wharton, C. (1992). Cognitive walkthroughs: A method for theory-based evaluation of user interfaces. *International Journal of Man–Machine Studies*, 36(5), 741–773. https://doi.org/10.1016/0020-7373(92)90039-N

Poole, A., & Ball, L. J. (2006). Eye tracking in HCI and usability research. In C. Ghaoui (Ed.), *Encyclopedia of Human–Computer Interaction* (pp. 211–219). IGI Global. https://doi.org/10.4018/978-1-59140-562-7.ch034

Pope, C., Halford, S., Turnbull, J., Prichard, J., Calestani, M., & May, C. (2013). Using computer decision support systems in NHS emergency and urgent care: Ethnographic study using normalisation process theory. *BMC Health Services Research*, 13, 111. https://doi.org/10.1186/1472-6963-13-111

Powers, E. M., Shiffman, R. N., Melnick, E. R., Hickner, A., & Sharifi, M. (2018). Efficacy and unintended consequences of hard-stop alerts in electronic health record systems: A systematic review. *Journal of the American Medical Informatics Association*, 25(11), 1556. https://doi.org/10.1093/jamia/ocy112

Preece, J. H., Rogers, Y., Sharp, H., Benyon, D., Holland, S., & Carey, T. (1994). *Human–computer interaction*. Addison-Wesley.

Preece, J., Rogers, Y., & Sharp, H. (2002). *Interaction design: Beyond human-computer interaction*. John Wiley & Sons.

Press, A., McCullagh, L., Khan, S., Schachter, A., Pardo, S., & McGinn, T. (2015). Usability testing of a complex clinical decision support tool in the emergency department: Lessons learned. *JMIR Human Factors*, 2(2), e14. https://doi.org/10.2196/humanfactors.4537

Protection of Human Research Subjects (2018). *45 U.S.C. § Part 46.401 exemptions*. Retrieved from www.hhs.gov/ohrp/regulations-and-policy/regulations/45-cfr-46/common-rule-subpart-a-46104/index.html

Protection of Human Research Subjects (2023). *45 U.S.C. § Part 46.116 General requirements for informed consent*. Retrieved from www.ecfr.gov/current/title-45/subtitle-A/subchapter-A/part-46

Punchoojit, L., & Hongwarittorrn, N. (2017). Usability studies on mobile user interface design patterns: A systematic literature review. *Advances in Human–Computer Interaction*, e6787504. https://doi.org/10.1155/2017/6787504

QSR International Ply Ltd. (n.d.). NVivo 12 qualitative data analysis software. *QSR International*. Retrieved from www.qsrinternational.com/nvivo/home

Qualtrics. (2023). *Qualtrics*. Retrieved from www.qualtrics.com

Rai, A., Chen, L., Pye, J., & Baird, A. (2013). Understanding determinants of consumer mobile health usage intentions, assimilation, and channel preferences. *Journal of Medical Internet Research*, 15(8), e149. https://doi.org/10.2196/jmir.2635

Ratzan, S. C., & Parker, R. M. (2000). Introduction. In C. R. Selden, M. Zorn, S. C. Ratzan, & R. M. Parker (Eds.), *National Library of Medicine current bibliographies in medicine: Health literacy* (pp. v–vi). National Institutes of Health.

Redish, G. (2010). Technical communication and usability: Intertwined strands and mutual influences. *IEEE Transactions on Professional Communication*, 53, 191–201. https://doi.org/10.1109/TPC.2010.2052861

Redish, J., & Lowry, S. Z. (2010). *Usability in health IT: Technical strategy, research, and implementation summary of workshop*. National Institute of Standards and Technology. https://doi.org/10.6028/NIST.IR.7743

Redish, J., Bias, R. G., Bailey, R., Molich, R., Dumas, J., & Spool, J. M. (2002). Usability in practice: Formative usability evaluations – evolution and revolution. In *CHI '02 Extended Abstracts on Human Factors in Computing Systems – CHI '02*, 885. https://doi.org/10.1145/506443.506647

Reeves, S., Kuper, A., & Hodges, B. D. (2008). Qualitative research methodologies: Ethnography. *BMJ Clinical Research*, 337, a1020. https://doi.org/10.1136/bmj.a1020

Resneck, J. S., Abrouk, M., Steuer, M., Tam, A., Yen, A., Lee, I., Kovarik, C. L., & Edison, K. E. (2016). Choice, transparency, coordination, and quality among direct-to-consumer telemedicine websites and apps treating skin disease. *JAMA Dermatology*, 152(7), 768. https://doi.org/10.1001/jamadermatol.2016.1774

Richardson, K. M., Fouquet, S. D., Kerns, E., & McCulloh, R. J. (2019). Impact of mobile device-based clinical decision support tool on guideline adherence and mental workload. *Academic Pediatrics*, 19(7), 828–834. https://doi.org/10.1016/j.acap.2019.03.001

Richardson, S., Mishuris, R., O'Connell, A., Feldstein, D., Hess, R., Smith, P., ... Mann, D. (2017). "Think aloud" and "near live" usability testing of two complex clinical decision support tools. *International Journal of Medical Informatics*, 106, 1–8.

Ritchie, J., & Lewis, J. (Eds.). (2003). *Qualitative research practice: A guide for social science students and researchers*. Sage.

Ritchie, J., & Spencer, L. (1994). Qualitative data analysis for applied policy research. In A. Bryman and R. G. Burgess (Eds.), *Analyzing qualitative data* (pp. 173–194). Routledge.

Rizvi, R. F., Marquard, J. L., Hultman, G. M., Adam, T. J., Harder, K. A., & Melton, G. B. (2017). Usability evaluation of electronic health record system around clinical notes usage: An ethnographic study. *Applied Clinical Informatics*, 8(4), 1095–1105. https://doi.org/10.4338/ACI-2017-04-RA-0067

Roche, T. R., Maas, E. J. C., Said, S., Braun, J., Machado, C., Spahn, D. R., Noethiger, C. B., & Tscholl, D. W. (2022). Anesthesia personnel's visual attention regarding patient monitoring in simulated non-critical and critical situations: An eye-tracking study. *BMC Anesthesiology*, 22(1), 167. https://doi.org/10.1186/s12871-022-01705-6

Rogers, M. L., Patterson, E., Chapman, R., & Render, M. (2005). Usability testing and the relation of clinical information systems to patient safety. In K. Henriksen, J. B. Battles, E. S. Marks, & D. I. Lewin (Eds.), *Advances in patient safety: From research to implementation (Vol. 2: Concepts and methodology)*. Agency for Healthcare Research and Quality. Retrieved from www.ncbi.nlm.nih.gov/books/NBK20503

Rosala, M. (2021, October 31). How many participants for a UX interview? Nielsen Norman Group. Retrieved from www.nngroup.com/articles/interview-sample-size

Rose, E. J. (2016). Design as advocacy: Using a human-centered approach to investigate the needs of vulnerable populations. *Journal of Technical Writing and Communication*, 46(4), 427–445. https://doi.org/10.1177/0047281616653494

Rose, E. J., Racadio, R., Wong, K., Nguyen, S., Kim, J., & Zahler, A. (2017). Community-Based User Experience: Evaluating the Usability of Health Insurance Information with Immigrant Patients. *IEEE Transactions on Professional Communication*, 60(2), 214–231. https://doi.org/10.1109/TPC.2017.2656698

Ruby, J. (1980). Exposing yourself: Reflexivity, anthropology, and film. *Semiotica*, 30(1–2), 153–180. https://doi.org/10.1515/semi.1980.30.1-2.153

Russ, A. L., & Saleem, J. J. (2018). Ten factors to consider when developing usability scenarios and tasks for health information technology. *Journal of Biomedical Informatics*, 78, 123–133.

Russ, A. L., Baker, D. A., Fahner, W. J., Milligan, B. S., Cox, L., Hagg, H. K., ... Saleem, J. J. (2010). A rapid usability evaluation (RUE) method for health information technology. In *AMIA 2010 Symposium Proceedings*, 702–706.

Sackett Catalogue of Bias Collaboration, Spencer, E. A., & Mahtani, K. (2017). Hawthorne effect. In *Catalogue of Bias 2017*. Retrieved from https://catalogofbias.org/biases/hawthorne-effect

Saitwal, H., Feng, X., Walji, M., Patel, V., & Zhang, J. (2010). Assessing performance of an electronic health record (EHR) using cognitive task analysis. *International Journal of Medical Informatics*, 79(7), 501–506. https://doi.org/10.1016/j.ijmedinf.2010.04.001

Sandefer, R. H., Westra, B. L., Khairat, S. S., Pieczkiewicz, D. S., & Speedie, S. M. (2015). Determinants of consumer eHealth information-seeking behavior. In *AMIA Annual Symposium Proceedings*, 1121–1129.

Sarkar, U., Gourley, G. I., Lyles, C. R., Tieu, L., Clarity, C., Newmark, L., Singh, K., & Bates, D. W. (2016). Usability of commercially available mobile applications for diverse patients. *Journal of General Internal Medicine*, 31(12), 1417–1426. https://doi.org/10.1007/s11606-016-3771-6

Sarkar, U., Karter, A. J., Liu, J. Y., Adler, N. E., Nguyen, R., López, A., & Schillinger, D. (2010). The literacy divide: Health literacy and the use of an internet-based patient portal in an integrated health system: Results from the Diabetes Study of Northern California (DISTANCE). *Journal of Health Communication*, 15(supp. 2), 183–196. https://doi.org/10.1080/10810730.2010.499988

Sauro, J. (2011, February 3). Measuring usability with the System Usability Scale (SUS). *MeasuringU*. Retrieved from https://measuringu.com/sus

Sauro, J. (2015, May 6). How to find the sample size for 8 common research designs. *MeasuringU*. Retrieved from https://measuringu.com/sample-size-designs

Sauro, J. (2018, September 19). 5 ways to interpret a SUS score. *MeasuringU*. Retrieved from https://measuringu.com/interpret-sus-score

Sauro, J. (2019, December 18). 10 things to know about the Post Study System Usability Questionnaire. *MeasuringU*. Retrieved from https://measuringu.com/pssuq/

Sauro, J., & Lewis, J. R. (2009). Correlations among prototypical usability metrics: Evidence for the construct of usability. In *Proceedings of the SIGCHI Conference on Human Factors in Computing Systems*, 1609–1618. https://doi.org/10.1145/1518701.1518947

Sauro, J., & Lewis, J. R. (2012). *Quantifying the user experience: Practical statistics for user research*. Elsevier/Morgan Kaufmann.

Sauro, J., & Lewis, J. R. (2016). *Quantifying the user experience: Practical statistics for user research* (2nd ed.). Elsevier/Morgan Kaufmann.

Sauro, J., & Lewis, J. R. (2023, January 27). Personal communication.

Sauro, J. & Lewis, J. R. (n.d.). *MeasuringU*. Retrieved from https://measuringu.com/calc

Schaaf, J., Prokosch, H.-U., Boeker, M., Schaefer, J., Vasseur, J., Storf, H., & Sedlmayr, M. (2020). Interviews with experts in rare diseases for the development of clinical decision support system software: A qualitative study. *BMC Medical Informatics and Decision Making*, 20, 230. https://doi.org/10.1186/s12911-020-01254-3

Schank, R. & Abelson, R. (1977). *Scripts, plans, goals and understanding: An inquiry into human knowledge structures*. Lawrence Erlbaum.

Schillewaert, N., Ahearne, M. J., Frambach, R. T., & Moenaert, R. K. (2005). The adoption of information technology in the sales force. *Industrial Marketing Management*, 34(4), 323–336.

Schmidt-Kraepelin, M., Dehling, T., & Sunyaev, A. (2014). Usability of patient-centered health IT: Mixed-methods usability study of ePill. *Studies in Health Technology and Informatics*, 198, 32–39. https://pubmed.ncbi.nlm.nih.gov/24825682/

Schnall, R., Cho, H., & Liu, J. (2018). Health Information Technology Usability Evaluation Scale (Health-ITUES) for usability assessment of mobile Health Technology: Validation Study. *JMIR MHealth and UHealth*, 6(1), e8851. https://doi.org/10.2196/mhealth.8851

Schoonenboom, J., & Johnson, R. B. (2017). How to construct a mixed methods research design. *Kolner Zeitschrift fur Soziologie und Sozialpsychologie*, 69(Suppl 2), 107–131. https://doi.org/10.1007/s11577-017-0454-1

Schumacher, R. M., & Lowry, S. Z. (2010). *NIST guide to the processes approach for improving the usability of electronic health records*. National Institute of Standards and Technology.

Scriven, M. (1967). The methodology of evaluation. In R.W. Tyler, R M. Gagne, & M. Scriven (eds.), *Perspectives of curriculum evaluation* (pp. 39–83). Rand McNally.

Shackel, B. (1981). The concept of usability. In *Proceedings of IBM Software and Information Usability Symposium*. IBM Corporation.

Shackel B. (1991). Usability context, framework, definition, design and evaluation. In B. Shackel, & S. J. Richardson (Eds.), *Human factors for informatics usability* (pp. 339–346). Cambridge University Press.

Shannon, C. E., & Weaver, W. (1998). *The mathematical theory of communication* (16th ed.). University of Illinois Press.

Sheehan, B., Nigrovic, L. E., Dayan, P. S., Kuppermann, N., Ballard, D. W., Alessandrini, E., … Bakken, S. (2013). Informing the design of clinical decision support services for evaluation of children with minor blunt head trauma in the emergency department: A sociotechnical analysis. *Journal of Biomedical Informatics*, 46(5), 905–913. https://doi.org/10.1016/j.jbi.2013.07.005

Shiffman, S., Stone, A. A., & Hufford, M. R. (2008). Ecological momentary assessment. *Annual Review of Clinical Psychology*, 4(1), 1–32. https://doi.org/10.1146/annurev.clinpsy.3.022 806.091415

Shneiderman, B. (1987). *Designing the user interface: Strategies for effective human–computer interaction*. Addison-Wesley.

Shneiderman, B., & Plaisant, C. (2010). *Designing the user interface* (5th ed.). Addison-Wesley.

Shuyler, K. S., & Knight, K. M. (2008). What are patients seeking when they turn to the internet? Qualitative content analysis of questions asked by visitors to an orthopaedics website. *Journal of Medical Internet Research*, 5(4), e24. https://doi.org/10.2196/jmir.5.4.e24

Silberg, W. M., Lundberg, G. D., & Musacchio, R. A. (1997). Assessing, controlling, and assuring the quality of medical information on the internet: Caveant Lector et Viewor—let the reader and viewer beware. *JAMA Network*, 277(15), 1244–1245.

Sillence, E., Briggs, P., Harris, P., & Fishwick, L. (2006). A framework for understanding trust factors in web-based health advice. *International Journal of Human–Computer Studies*, 64(8), 697–713. https://doi.org/10.1016/j.ijhcs.2006.02.007

Slife, B. D., & Gantt, E. E. (1999). Methodological pluralism: A framework for psychotherapy research. *Journal of Clinical Psychology*, 55(12), 1453–1465. https://doi.org/10.1002/(SICI)1097-4679(199912)55:12<1453::AID-JCLP4>3.0.CO;2-C

Sloan, M., Lever, E., Harwood, R., Gordon, C., Wincup, C., Blane, M., Brimicombe, J., Lanyon, P., Howard, P., Sutton, S., D'Cruz, D., & Naughton, F. (2022). Telemedicine in rheumatology: A mixed methods study exploring acceptability, preferences and experiences among patients and clinicians. *Rheumatology*, 61(6), 2262–2274. https://doi.org/10.1093/rheumatology/keab796

Slovic, P. (1982). Toward understanding and improving decisions. In W. C. Howell & E. A. Fleishman (Eds.), *Human performance and productivity: Vol. 2—Information processing and decision making* (pp. 157–183). Lawrence Erlbaum.

Sousa, V. E. C., & Dunn Lopez, K. (2017). Towards usable e-Health: A systematic review of usability questionnaires. *Applied Clinical Informatics*, 8(2), 470–490. https://doi.org/10.4338/ACI-2016-10-R-0170

Sousa, V. E. C., & Lopez, K. D. (2017). Towards usable e-Health. *Applied Clinical Informatics*, 8(2), 470–490. https://doi.org/10.4338/ACI-2016-10-R-0170

Spinuzzi, C. (2005). The methodology of participatory design. *Technical Communication*, 52(2), 163–174.

Srivastava, A., & Thomson, S. B. (2009). Framework analysis: A qualitative methodology for applied policy research. *Journal of Administration and Governance*, 4(2), 72–79.

St.Amant, K. (2017). The cultural context of care in international communication design: A heuristic for addressing usability in international health and medical communication. *Communication Design Quarterly*, 5(2), 62–70.

St.Amant, K. (2018). Culture, context, and usability. *Intercom*, May/June, 31–32.

St.Amant, K. (2020). Cognition, care, and usability: Applying cognitive concepts to user experience design in health and medical contexts. *Journal of Technical Writing and Communication*, 004728162098156. https://doi.org/10.1177/0047281620981567

St.Amant, K. (2021). Context, cognition, and communication: Understanding how the psychology of location affects health and medical communication. *European Scientific Journal*, 17(30), 8. https://doi.org/10.19044/esj.2021.v17n30p8

Stanton, N. A., Salmon, P. M., Rafferty, L. A., Walker, G. H., Baber, C., & Jenkins, D. P. (2017). *Human factors methods: A practical guide for engineering and design*. CRC Press.

Stemler, S. (2001). An overview of content analysis. *Practical Assessment, Research, and Evaluation*, 7(17). https://doi.org/10.7275/z6fm-2e34

Subedi, K. R. (2021). Determining the sample in qualitative research. *Scholars' Journal*, 1–13. https://doi.org/10.3126/scholars.v4i1.42457

Sun, Y., Zhang, Y., Gwizdka, J., & Trace, C. B. (2019). Consumer evaluation of the quality of online health information: Systematic Literature Review of Relevant Criteria and Indicators. *Journal of Medical Internet Research*, 21(5), e12522. https://doi.org/10.2196/12522

SurveyMonkey. (2023). *SurveyMonkey by momentive*. Retrieved from www.surveymonkey.com

T. W. (n. d.). Measuring and interpreting System Usability Scale (SUS). *UIUX Trend*. Retrieved from https://uiuxtrend.com/measuring-system-usability-scalesus/#interpretation

Takahashi, L., & Nebe, K. (2019). Observed differences between lab and online tests using the AttrakDiff Semantic Differential Scale. *The Journal of User Experience*, 14(2), 65–75. Retrieved from https://uxpajournal.org/attrakdiff-semantic-differential-scale

Tang, Y., Yang, Y.-T., & Shao, Y.-F. (2019). Acceptance of online medical websites: An empirical study in China. *International Journal of Environmental Research and Public Health*, 16(6), 943. https://doi.org/10.3390/ijerph16060943

tobii. (2022). tobii. Retrieved from www.tobii.com

Tognazzini, B. (2014, March 6). First principles of interaction design. *AskTog*. Retrieved from https://asktog.com/atc/principles-of-interaction-design

Tomkins, S. S. (1962). *Affect imagery consciousness. Volume 1: The Positive Affects*. Springer.

Tomkins, S. S. (1987). Script theory. In J. Aronoff, A. I. Rabin, & R. A. Zucker (Eds.), *The emergence of personality* (pp. 147–216). Springer.

Travis, D. (2009, October 5). How to prioritise usability problems. *Userfocus*. Retrieved from www.userfocus.co.uk/articles/prioritise.html

Tuckson, R. V., Edmunds, M., & Hodgkins, M. L. (2017). Telehealth. *The New England Journal of Telemedicine*, 377, 1585–1592. https://doi.org/10.1056/NEJMsr1503323

Tullis, T. S., & Stetson, J. N. (2004). A comparison of questionnaires for assessing website usability. *Proceedings of UPA: Usability Professionals' Association Conference 2004*.

Twohig, I. (2022, September 5). Tips for using a diary study for patient experience research. *Indeemo*. Retrieved from https://indeemo.com/blog/diary-study-for-patient-experience-research

U.S. Department of Health and Human Services (HHS). (n.d.). Research-Based Web Design and Usability Guidelines. Washington, D.C.: U.S. Department of Health and Human Services (HHS) and the U.S. General Services Administration (GSA): Government Printing Office. Retrieved from https://guidelines.usability.gov/

University of Maryland UM Ventures. (1999, March 9). *QUIS™—the Questionnaire for User Interaction Satisfaction*. University of Maryland. Retrieved from www.umventures.org/technologies/quis%E2%84%A2-questionnaire-user-interaction-satisfaction-0

Uscher-Pines, L., & Mehrotra, A. (2014). Analysis of teladoc use seems to indicate expanded access to care for patients without prior connection to a provider. *Health Affairs*, 33(2), 258–264. https://doi.org/10.1377/hlthaff.2013.0989

Uscher-Pines, L., Mulcahy, A., Cowling, D., Hunter, G., Burns, R., & Mehrotra, A. (2015). Antibiotic prescribing for acute respiratory infections in direct-to-consumer telemedicine visits. *JAMA Internal Medicine*, 175(7), 1234. https://doi.org/10.1001/jamaintern med.2015.2024

Uscher-Pines, L., Mulcahy, A., Cowling, D., Hunter, G., Burns, R., & Mehrotra, A. (2016). Access and quality of care in direct-to-consumer telemedicine. *Telemedicine and e-Health*, 22(4), 282–287. https://doi.org/10.1089/tmj.2015.0079

van Osch, M., Rövekamp, A., Bergman-Agteres, S. N., Wijsman, L. W., Ooms, S. J., Mooijaart, S. P., & Vermeulen, J. (2015). User preferences and usability of iVitality: Optimizing an innovative online research platform for home-based health monitoring. *Patient Preference and Adherence*, 9, 857–867. https://doi.org/10.2147/PPA.S82510

van Someren, M. W., Barnard, Y. F., & Sandberg, J. A. C. (1994). *The think aloud method: A practical guide to modeling cognitive processes*. Academic Press.

Vasileiou, K., Barnett, J., Thorpe, S., & Young, T. (2018). Characterising and justifying sample size sufficiency in interview-based studies: Systematic analysis of qualitative health research over a 15-year period. *BMC Medical Research Methodology*, 18(1), 148. https://doi.org/10.1186/s12874-018-0594-7

Vaske, J. J. (2002). Communicating judgments about practical significance: Effect size, confidence intervals and odds ratios. *Human Dimensions of Wildlife*, 7(4), 287–300. https://doi.org/10.1080/10871200214752

Velazquez, C. E., & Pasch, K. E. (2014). Attention to food and beverage advertisements as measured by eye-tracking technology and the food preferences and choices of youth. *Journal of the Academy of Nutrition and Dietetics*, 114(4), 578–582. https://doi.org/10.1016/j.jand.2013.09.030

Venkatesh, V., Brown, S. A., & Bala, H. (2013). Bridging the qualitative–quantitative divide: Guidelines for conducting mixed methods research in information systems. *MIS Quarterly*, 37(1), 21–54. https://doi.org/10.25300/MISQ/2013/37.1.02

Virzi, R. (1992). Refining the test phase of usability evaluation: How many subjects is enough? *Human Factors Society*, 34: 457–468.

Visweswaran, S., King, A. J., Tajgardoon, M., Calzoni, L., Clermont, G., Hochheiser, H., & Cooper, G. F. (2021). Evaluation of eye tracking for a decision support application. *JAMIA Open*, 4(3), ooab059. https://doi.org/10.1093/jamiaopen/ooab059

Weinsc Inostroza, R., Rusu, C., Roncagliolo, S., Jimenez, C., & Rusu, V. (2012). Usability heuristics for touchscreen-based mobile devices. *2012 Ninth International Conference on Information Technology—New Generations*, 662–667. https://doi.org/10.1109/ITNG.2012.134

Weinschenk, S. & Barker, D. (2000). *Designing effective speech interfaces*. Wiley.

Weiss, B. D. (2003). *Health literacy: A manual for clinicians*. American Medical Association Foundation and American Medical Association.

Weiss, E. (1993). *Making computers people-literate*. Jossey-Bass.

Wharton, C., Rieman, J., Lewis, C., Polson, P. (1994). The cognitive walkthrough method: A practitioner's guide. In J. Nielsen, & R. L. Mack (Eds.), *Usability inspection methods* (pp. 105–139). John Wiley & Sons.

White, M. D., & Marsh, E. E. (2006). Content analysis: A flexible methodology. *Library Trends*, 55(1), 22–45. https://doi.org/10.1353/lib.2006.0053

Whitehead, H., May, D., & Agahi, H. (2007). An exploratory study into the factors that influence patients' perceptions of cleanliness in an acute NHS trust hospital. *Journal of Facilities Management*, 5(4), 275–289.

Whiteside, J., Bennett, J., & Holtzblatt, K. (1988). Usability engineering: Our experience and evolution. In J. Vanderdonckt, P. Palanque, & M. Winckler (Eds.), *Handbook of Human–Computer Interaction* (pp. 791–817). Elsevier. https://doi.org/10.1016/B978-0-444-70536-5.50041-5

Whitten, P., Johannessen, L. K., Soerensen, T., Gammon, D., & Mackert, M. (2007). A systematic review of research methodology in telemedicine studies. *Journal of Telemedicine and Telecare*, 13(5), 230–235. https://doi.org/10.1258/135763307781458976

Wildemuth, B. M. (Ed.). (2017). *Applications of social research methods to questions in information and library science* (2nd ed.). Libraries Unlimited.

Willis, M., Brand Hein, L., Hu, Z., Saran, R., Argentina, M., Bragg-Gresham, J., Krein, S. L., Gillespie, B., Zheng, K., & Veinot, T. C. (2021). Usability evaluation of a tablet-based intervention to prevent intradialytic hypotension in dialysis patients during in-clinic dialysis: Mixed methods study. *JMIR Human Factors*, 8(2), e26012. https://doi.org/10.2196/26012

Wilson, E. V. (Ed.). (2009). *Patient-centered e-health*. IGI Global.

Wilson, F. L., Racine, E., Tekieli, V., & Williams, B. (2003). Literacy, readability and cultural barriers: Critical factors to consider when educating older African Americans about anticoagulation therapy. *Journal of Clinical Nursing*, 12(2), 275–282.

Winter, G. (2000). A comparative discussion of the notion of validity in qualitative and quantitative research. *The Qualitative Report*, 4(3), 1–14. https://doi.org/10.46743/2160-3715/2000.2078

Wolpin, S., Halpenny, B., Whitman, G., McReynolds, J., Stewart, M., Lober, W., & Berry, D. (2015). Development and usability testing of a web-based cancer symptom and quality-of-life support intervention. *Health Informatics Journal*, 21(1), 10–23. https://doi.org/10.1177/1460458213495744

Woodruff, A., Faulring, A., Rosenholtz, R., Morrsion, J., & Pirolli, P. (2001). Using thumbnails to search the web. In *Proceedings of the SIGCHI Conference on Human Factors in Computing Systems*, 198–205. https://doi.org/10.1145/365024.365098

Wronikowska, M. W., Malycha, J., Morgan, L. J., Westgate, V., Petrinic, T., Young, J. D., & Watkinson, P. J. (2021). Systematic review of applied usability metrics within usability evaluation methods for hospital electronic healthcare record systems: Metrics and evaluation methods for eHealth systems. *Journal of Evaluation in Clinical Practice*, 27(6), 1403–1416. https://doi.org/10.1111/jep.13582

Xie, B., Zhou, J., & Wang, H. (2017). How influential are mental models on interaction performance? Exploring the gap between users' and designers' mental models through a new quantitative method. *Advances in Human–Computer Interaction*, 1–14. https://doi.org/10.1155/2017/3683546

Yang, S.-N., & McConkie, G. W. (2001). Eye movements during reading: A theory of saccade initiation times. *Vision Research*, 41(25), 3567–3585. https://doi.org/10.1016/S0042-6989(01)00025-6

Yen, P. Y., & Bakken, S. (2012). Review of health information technology usability study methodologies. *Journal of the American Medical Informatics Association*, 19(3), 413–422. https://doi.org/10.1136/amiajnl-2010-000020

Yen, P.-Y., McAlearney, A. S., Sieck, C. J., Hefner, J. L., & Huerta, T. R. (2017). Health information technology (HIT) adaptation: Refocusing on the journey to successful HIT implementation. *JMIR Medical Informatics*, 5(3), e28. https://doi.org/10.2196/medinform.7476

Yip, M. P., Chang, A. M., Chan, J., & MacKenzie, A. E. (2003). Development of the Telemedicine Satisfaction Questionnaire to evaluate patient satisfaction with telemedicine: A preliminary study. *Journal of Telemedicine and Telecare*, 9(1), 46–50. https://doi.org/10.1258/135763303321159693

Youssef, N., Ghazy, R. M., Mahdy, R. E., Abdalgabar, M., Elshaarawy, O., & Alboraie, M. (2022). Development, validity, and reliability of the perceived Telemedicine Importance,

Disadvantages, and Barriers (PTIDB) Questionnaire for Egyptian healthcare professionals. *International Journal of Environmental Research and Public Health*, 19(19), 12678. https://doi.org/10.3390/ijerph191912678

Zapf, A., Castell, S., Morawietz, L., & Karch, A. (2016). Measuring inter-rater reliability for nominal data: Which coefficients and confidence intervals are appropriate? *BMC Medical Research Methodology*, 16, 93. https://doi.org/10.1186/s12874-016-0200-9

Zhang, J., Johnson, T. R., Patel, V. L., Paige, D. L., & Kubose, T. (2003). Using usability heuristics to evaluate patient safety of medical devices. *Journal of Biomedical Informatics*, 36(1–2), 23–30. https://doi.org/10.1016/S1532-0464(03)00060-1

Zhang, J., & Walji, M. F. (2011). TURF: Toward a unified framework of EHR usability. *Journal of Biomedical Informatics*, 44(6), 1056–1067. https://doi.org/10.1016/j.jbi.2011.08.005

Zhang, L., Babu, S. V., Jindal, M., Williams, J. E., & Gimbel, R. W. (2019). A patient-centered mobile phone app (iHeartU) with a virtual human assistant for self-management of heart failure: Protocol for a usability assessment study. *JMIR Research Protocols*, 8(5), e13502. https://doi.org/10.2196/13502

Zhang, S., Brown, T., Weiss, S., Ruvalcaba, E., David, M., Boorman, E., Lanzkron, S. M., & Eakin, M. (2021). Telemedicine has acceptable usability and high satisfaction in patients with sickle cell disease. *Blood*, 138, 2982. https://doi.org/10.1182/blood-2021-149111

Zolnoori, M., Balls-Berry, J. E., Brockman, T. A., Patten, C. A., Huang, M., & Yao, L. (2019). A systematic framework for analyzing patient-generated narrative data: Protocol for a content analysis. *JMIR Research Protocols*, 8(8), e13914. https://doi.org/10.2196/13914

Zulman, D. M., Jenchura, E. C., Cohen, D. M., Lewis, E. T., Houston, T. K., & Asch, S. M. (2015). How can eHealth technology address challenges related to multimorbidity? Perspectives from patients with multiple chronic conditions. *Journal of General Internal Medicine*, 30(8), 1063–1070. https://doi.org/10.1007/s11606-015-3222-9

Appendix A

Sample Informed Consent Form

| Insert Institution Logo Here |

TITLE OF RESEARCH STUDY: [INSERT TEXT HERE]

Investigator: [*Insert text here*]

<u>*Key Information:*</u> The following is a short summary of this study to help you decide whether or not to be a part of this study. More detailed information is listed later on in this form.

Why am I being invited to take part in a research study?

We invite you take part in this research study because *Insert text here.*

Why is this research being done?

This research is being performed because *Insert text here.*

How long will the research last and what will I need to do?

Insert text here.

Is there any way being in this study could be bad for me?

The risks of participation are minimal and do not exceed the risks associated with the activities performed in daily life.

Will being in this study help me any way?

Insert text here.

What happens if I do not want to be in this research?

Participation in research is completely voluntary. You can decide to participate or not to participate. You are free to withdraw your consent and discontinue participation in this study at any time without prejudice or penalty. Your decision to participate or not participate in this study will in no way affect your *Insert text here if applicable.*

Detailed Information: The following is more detailed information about this study in addition to the information listed above.

What should I know about a research study?

- Someone will explain this research study to you.
- Whether or not you take part is up to you.
- You can choose not to take part.
- You can agree to take part and later change your mind.
- Your decision will not be held against you.
- You can ask all the questions you want before you decide.

Who can I talk to?

If you have questions, concerns, or complaints, or think the research has hurt you, please contact the primary researcher, *Insert text here.*

This research has been reviewed and approved by an Institutional Review Board ("IRB"). You may talk to them at *Insert text here* if:

- Your questions, concerns, or complaints are not being answered by the research team.
- You cannot reach the research team.
- You want to talk to someone besides the research team.
- You have questions about your rights as a research subject.
- You want to get information or provide input about this research.

How many people will be studied?

We expect *Insert text here* people will be in this research study.

What happens if I say yes, I want to be in this research?

If you decide to participate in this research study, the primary researcher *Insert text here*.

To participate in the study, you will be required to be at least 18 years of age and *Insert text here*.

The following is a description of what will occur during your usability testing session.

1. The primary researcher will describe the purpose of the study and the study protocol.
2. She will confirm that you understand the study, agree to participate, and gain your signed consent to participate in the study.
3. You will be asked to provide demographics, such as your gender, age, where you are from, and previous use of telemedicine.
4. You will be provided a written and verbal description of an artificial scenario, in which you are ill and looking for medical care.
5. You will be asked to *Insert text here*.

What happens if I say yes, but I change my mind later?

You can leave the research at any time and it will not be held against you. If you decide to stop participating, let the primary researcher know during the study.

What happens to the information collected for the research?

Efforts will be made to limit the use and disclosure of your personal information, including the data gained as a result of your participation, to only people who have a need to review the information. We cannot promise complete secrecy. The *Insert text here* IRB may inspect and copy your information. Your name and contact information will be used to schedule the usability test, and the information will not be released elsewhere. Your demographic information may be included in publication of the results and will not be associated with your name. Please ask the primary researcher for more details if you have privacy and confidentiality concerns. If you agree to take part in this research study, you will be rewarded with a *Insert text here* for your time and effort.

If you understand the information in this document and consent to participate in this research study, please print and sign your name and date on the next two pages. You will be given one of the signed permission forms to take with you, and one will be retained for purposes of the study.

Your signature documents your permission to take part in this research.

_____   _____
Signature of subject   Date

_____
Printed name of subject

_____   _____
Signature of person obtaining consent   Date

_____
Printed name of person obtaining consent

Your signature documents your permission to take part in this research.

_____   _____
Signature of subject   Date

_____
Printed name of subject

_____   _____
Signature of person obtaining consent   Date

_____
Printed name of person obtaining consent

Appendix B

System Usability Scale (SUS)

Change the word "system" to whatever term best suits the artifact the participants interacted with/the artifact under investigation (for example, "website," "application," "product," "device").

Please indicate your level of agreement or disagreement with the following statements about your experience interacting with the system using the five-point Likert scale.

	Statement	1 Strongly disagree	2 Disagree	3 Neither agree nor disagree	4 Agree	5 Strongly agree
1	I think that I would like to use this system frequently.					
2	I found the system unnecessarily complex.					
3	I thought the system was easy to use.					
4	I think that I would need the support of a technical person to be able to use this system.					
5	I found the various functions in this system were well integrated.					
6	I thought there was too much inconsistency in this system.					
7	I would imagine that most people would learn to use this system very quickly.					
8	I found the system very cumbersome to use.					

	Statement	1 Strongly disagree	2 Disagree	3 Neither agree nor disagree	4 Agree	5 Strongly agree
9	I felt very confident using the system.					
10	I needed to learn a lot of things before I could get going with this system.					

Appendix C

Quick Reference Sheet for Study Sample Sizes for Common UX Research Methods

Please note that the sample size numbers offered in the table below are synthesized from experiential knowledge and industry best practices. Every study is unique and has various circumstances that will implicate the determination of your sample size.

UX research method	Sample size	Research objective
Ethnography	Depends on context (0-many)	To generate overall understanding of phenomenon within context (qualitative insights)
Contextual inquiry	Depends on depth/time (10–12)	To gain an in-depth understanding of users and context (qualitative insights)
Interview	5–10 per user group	To create user personas (UX artifact)
	10–12	To generate overall understanding of phenomenon (qualitative insights)
	20–30	To be able to draw comparisons and make generalizations
Survey	100	To make generalizations
Diary studies	6–12	To gain rich detail of a user journey
	30–60	To gain an understanding of the breadth of themes across user journeys
Heuristic evaluation	3 double experts or 5 experts	To be able to identify about 80 percent of the usability problems

UX research method	Sample size	Research objective
Cognitive Walkthrough	3 double experts or 5 experts	To be able to identify about 80 percent of the usability problems
Think-aloud usability testing	5	To be able to identify about 85 percent of the usability problems
Quantitative usability testing	20	To be able to generate statistically significant results
Questionnaires and scales (SUS)	100	To be able to generalize results

Index

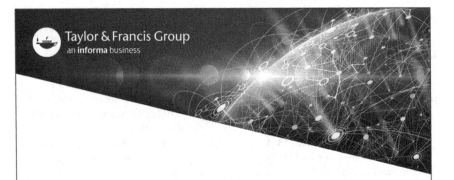

Printed in the United States
by Baker & Taylor Publisher Services